T0174451

Remington Education

Physical Pharmacy

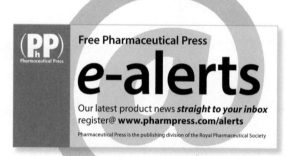

Free Pharmaceutical Press

e-alerts

Our latest product news *straight to your inbox*
register@ **www.pharmpress.com/alerts**

Pharmaceutical Press is the publishing division of the Royal Pharmaceutical Society

Remington Education

Physical Pharmacy

Blaine T Smith RPh, PhD

Pharmaceutical Press

Published by Pharmaceutical Press

66–68 East Smithfield, London E1W 1AW

© The Royal Pharmaceutical Society 2016

(**P.P**) is a trade mark of Pharmaceutical Press

Pharmaceutical Press is the publishing division of the Royal Pharmaceutical Society

Typeset by Swales & Willis Ltd, Exeter, Devon, UK
Printed in Great Britain by TJ International, Padstow, Cornwall

ISBN 978 0 85711 106 7
epdf 978 0 85711 252 1
ePub 978 0 85711 253 8
mobi 978 0 85711 254 5

All rights reserved. No part of this publication may be reproduced, stored in a retrieval system, or transmitted in any form or by any means, without the prior written permission of the copyright holder.

The publisher makes no representation, express or implied, with regard to the accuracy of the information contained in this book and cannot accept any legal responsibility or liability for any errors or omissions that may be made.

The rights of Blaine T Smith to be identified as the author of this work have been asserted by him in accordance with the Copyright, Designs and Patents Act 1988.

A catalogue record for this book is available from the British Library.

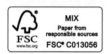

MIX
Paper from
responsible sources
FSC
www.fsc.org FSC® C013056

Contents

Preface

This book was written with the intent of providing a supplement for students of pharmacy and pharmaceutics to reinforce many of the basic principles of physical pharmacy, as they relate to drug delivery systems. It should be helpful to those looking for additional reading for their studies, as a text for physical pharmacy topics as they are presented with professional pharmacy curricula, and as a reference for those wishing to study certain topics presented in an alternative fashion to that provided in the classroom.

It is often helpful to study a text that parallels or reinforces materials studied in a course, perhaps presented with a different approach than that used in the classroom, such that meanings and emphases regarding the topic can be reinforced. Use of this text by those teaching physical pharmacy will provide an easy means of presenting a physical pharmacy standalone course or a section of physical pharmacy integrated into an overarching pharmaceutics course. This book is not intended to be an exhaustive discourse of physical pharmacy. It is intended to bring out the basic concepts that can be applied to more complex situations, providing a background based on the underlying physics and chemistry that dictate the actions of dosage forms and their components.

By providing a simple introduction to the topic of physical pharmacy, it is hoped the trepidation of many students can be alleviated, and the topic will not end up as daunting to master as one may imagine, as the course looms ahead in the curriculum. Key points are highlighted in order to easily orient the reader to the text and to provide a quick reference.

Pharmaceutics involves all aspects of the drug delivery system that pertain to its composition and performance. Physical pharmacy is the subcategory focusing on the reasons that drug delivery systems behave as they do. In order for pharmacists and formulators to understand, predict and provide optimally useful drug delivery systems, the pertinent aspects of physical pharmacy should be a routine consideration.

Blaine T Smith RPh, PhD
May, 2015

About the author

Blaine Templar Smith earned his Bachelor's degrees in Chemistry and Pharmacy and a PhD in Pharmaceutical Sciences (with emphasis in Nuclear Pharmacy and Immunology) at the University of Oklahoma. Dr Smith is a Registered Pharmacist in both Oklahoma and Massachusetts, practicing in a very wide spectrum of settings, including hospital inpatient, long-term care centers, independent and chain retail pharmacies, and Indian Health Service clinics and hospitals. He completed a postdoctoral fellowship at the University of Oklahoma Genome Sequencing Center, participating in the Human Genome Project.

Dr Smith has been a faculty member at the University of Oklahoma College of Pharmacy, the Massachusetts College of Pharmacy and Health Sciences-Worcester, a faculty member and chair of the Department of Pharmaceutical Sciences at the Saint Joseph University School of Pharmacy and a visiting fellow at the University of Massachusetts Medical School.

He has written, edited and published reference and textbooks related to the fields of medicine, pharmacy, pharmaceutics, physical pharmacy, nuclear pharmacy, immunology, molecular biology, diagnostic imaging and nursing. Additionally, he provides both written and online (live and asynchronous) continuing education, for health care professionals.

Acknowledgments

Table 1.3 is reprinted from P. Schwerdtfeger, 'Atomic Static Dipole Polarizabilities', in *Computational Aspects of Electric Polarizability Calculations: Atoms, Molecules and Clusters,* ed. G. Maroulis, IOS Press, Amsterdam, 2006; pp. 1–32. 'Table of experimental and calculated static dipole polarizabilities for the electronic ground states of the neutral elements (in atomic units)'. Updated static dipole polarizabilities are available as a PDF file from the Center for Theoretical Chemistry and Physics (CTCP) website at Massey University: http://ctcp.massey.ac.nz/Tablepol2014.pdf (accessed 6 June 2015). Also from *Transport Properties of Ions in Gases*, Appendix III 'Tables of Properties Useful in the Estimation of Ionneutral Interaction Energies', pp. 531–539, Wiley Online Library, 28 Jan 2005.

Table 4.3 is reprinted from *Remington* 22nd edn, Appendix A 'Sodium Chloride Equivalents, Freezing Point Depressions, and Hemolytic Effects of Certain Medicinals in Aqueous Solution', pp. 652–664 (ISBN 978 0 85711 062 6 [print = ISSN 1558 2922]).

Table 4.6 is reprinted from *Remington* 21st edn, Appendix B 'Isotonic Solution V-Values', p. 265.

Table 5.2 is reprinted from *Remington* 21st edn, 'HLB Values of Common Emulsifiers Used in Pharmaceutical Systems', p. 760, Table 39.6.

Figure 3.3 is taken from *FastTrack*, Figure 2.2.

Figure 3.11 is taken from *FastTrack*, Figure 1.4.

Figure 6.1 is taken from *Chemistry: The Central Science,* Chapter 13, Section 6, Figure 13.25.

http://wps.prenhall.com/wps/media/objects/3082/3156628/blb1306.html (accessed 6 June 2015).

Figure 6.2 is taken from *Chemistry: The Central Science,* Chapter 13, Section 6, Figure 13.29.

http://wps.prenhall.com/wps/media/objects/3082/3156628/blb1306.html (accessed 6 June 2015).

Figure 7.11 is taken from *Remington* 22nd edn, p. 745, Figure 36.6.

Introduction

What is physical pharmacy? It is the study of the influences of physics and chemistry on drug dosage forms, and the study of the effects dosage forms have on their environment. The emphasis of physical pharmacy is the physical characteristics and actions dosage forms (drug delivery systems) possess, mainly before the dosage form is given to the patient. The physical characteristics and actions of all drug delivery systems are dictated predominantly by intermolecular interactions. Intermolecular interactions, in turn, are governed by the laws of physics and chemistry. Some drug delivery systems behave the way they do because of the actions of electrostatic attraction and repulsion among their components. Other drug delivery systems depend on general physical characteristics, chemical reactions, or the simple rules of physics, such as relative hydrophilicity or hydrophobicity. Understanding the bases on which drug delivery systems 'work' will enable the reader to predict physical attributes and potential problems that the use of a particular dosage form may present. However, understanding the underlying causes and effects of physics and chemistry on dosage forms will enable the reader to intelligently manipulate dosage forms, optimize conditions under which the best results for drug therapy may be obtained, and then create the most stable and elegant delivery systems for particular needs. Understanding and advantageous utilization of the effectors of dosage forms are the goals of physical pharmacy.

In order to achieve optimal drug delivery to a patient, the appropriate drug form must be used. The patient may receive sub-optimal (or more costly) therapeutic benefits from a given drug if it is not provided in a dosage form that promotes ideal delivery. The proper dosage form and its detailed design, in turn, depend on the selective application of the physical and chemical attributes of the drug, the delivery system, and patient physiology. Being mindful of the laws governing these areas allows the best and most consistent delivery of drugs to patients.

But drug delivery is the final step where physical pharmacy is involved. Physical pharmacy contributes to the steps preceding the successful delivery of drugs to their targets. A drug must be stable within the selected dosage form, free from any chemical or physical changes caused by the components of the delivery system, and from the effects of the storage environment. The drug – and its delivery system – should remain unchanged during storage: the characteristic of a drug and its delivery to a patient must be predictable the day of its manufacture or compounding, and after periods of shipping and storage, which may occur before drug administration.

Alterations in temperature, agitation or shaking, and the amount of time elapsed since manufacture must be endured by the drug product, while still retaining the required consistency in physical and chemical attributes and therapeutic effect.

Effectors of dosage form longevity

The lifespan of a dosage form depends on many variables, some of which can be controlled or accounted for and some of which cannot. Examples of the controllable variables include the characteristics and parameters of diffusion, electrostatic attraction and repulsion, settling due to gravity, separation of components due to incompatibility, or chemical or physical phenomena, improper aggregation of particles, changes in particle size, and the effects of the environment, such as temperature fluctuations.

An understanding of the obstacles to drug delivery, such as those simply involving entropy, is helpful. It is often difficult, if not impossible, to successfully compensate for all obstacles and still retain the ability to formulate a proper drug delivery system. However, thoughtful compensation or prevention of important impediments to drug delivery may well be possible. So it is prudent to study and understand the factors that affect drugs and dosage forms. Therefore, we can at least understand the limitations of specific drug delivery systems.

Ultimately, we can design systems that are stable for great periods of time and ensure safe, optimum, and effective delivery of drugs to their sites of action. For those responsible for the safe-keeping, dispensing, and administration of drug delivery systems, the understanding of physical pharmacy will enable proper handling, storage, and administration of dosage forms – not blindly, with the hope that all was proper, but with the confidence that stems from knowing everything possible was done to ensure patient responses that are dependent on drug delivery systems are the best possible.

Patient variability

There will probably always be variability in patient responses to drugs. This variability should not be due to aspects of the dosage form, but rather to inter-patient biological and/or genetic differences. Beyond the parameters of drug delivery related to physical pharmacy are those pertaining to the patient. This is where the biopharmaceutics, pharmacogenetics, and pharmacogenomics of patient responses become important.

The focus of this text will be on the factors and phenomena of drug delivery systems that may be encountered from creation to delivery of the drugs to their targets. There is some overlap between biopharmaceutics and physical pharmacy as the spectrum of study proceeds, but the intent of the writing of this book is to adhere mainly to aspects normally considered within the domain of physical pharmacy.

The drug delivery system

As previously stated, the types of issues that are addressed by physical pharmacy have their bases on the molecular level. Drug delivery systems often are composed of several components, each added for a specific purpose. These components will necessarily interact with themselves and each other on a molecular level. These interactions can either be necessary or, as is most often the case, inconsequential to the ultimate action of the active component (drug). How these components interact with each other can have a bearing on the success or failure of the drug delivery systems. Molecular interactions of most concern to us involve forces of attraction and repulsion between regions of molecules. When viewed more macroscopically, these attractive and repulsive actions directly affect solubility, dissolution rate, behavior of solids, liquids, gasses, as well as the general characteristics of solutions and dispersions. Particle diffusion and stable dispersion of insoluble particles, such as colloids, suspensions, and emulsions, are based on how their molecules interact with each other. The molecular interactions – positive or negative (attractive or repulsive) – can be intentionally used to produce a desired delivery system. Not all repulsive interactions are inherently detrimental, nor are all attractive forces innately beneficial. It is these thoughtful, judicious applications that we strive for.

What can we control?

Can we manipulate solubility and dissolution rate? If so, why would we want to do this? How can we knowingly make particles repel each other and why should this even be beneficial for drug delivery? Can we keep liquid drug delivery systems from settling to the bottoms of their containers over time and thus improve dosage form reliability? How can we deliver drugs by mouth that otherwise would taste bad? How can we 'dissolve' a hydrophobic drug in an aqueous medium? Can it be predicted if a particular solid will actually dissolve in a vehicle? When drugs are administered parenterally it is especially important to be cognizant of maintaining tonicity, or osmotic pressure. How can we ensure tonicity is maintained so that cell or tissue damage does not occur? If we mix hydrophilic and hydrophobic compounds together, what will happen? Can we change the outcome? Can we predict whether we can add something to a drug delivery system without destabilizing it? Can we use temperature fluctuations to our advantage or can we preclude the adverse consequences that temperature fluctuations may have on drug delivery systems?

What is the difference between physical pharmacy and pharmaceutics? Physical pharmacy is included in the more general area of pharmaceutics. Pharmaceutics is the science of drug delivery system preparation and use and includes Physical Pharmacy, Biopharmaceutics, and Pharmacokinetics. Physical pharmacy is the study of/application of physics and chemistry as they pertain to drug delivery systems.

1

Intermolecular interactions

Learning objectives

Upon completion of this chapter, you should be able to answer the following questions:

- What are intermolecular interactions?
- Why are electrostatic interactions in liquids important?
- What roles do cohesive and adhesive forces play in the mixing and separation of liquids?
- What is polarity?
- What is a dipole moment?
- What is an induced dipole?
- Why are dipoles important for solubility?
- What effect does individual atomic electronegativity have on solubility?
- Why do liquids deviate from the Ideal Gas law?
- What factors exert the greatest influences on intermolecular interactions?

Intermolecular interactions

Intermolecular interactions – those between molecules – dictate much of the physical characteristics of the world around us. When analyzed, intermolecular interactions originate from intramolecular interactions – those within molecules. Though the effects of intermolecular interactions can be seen in all physical phases (solid, liquid, gas), perhaps the most important for pharmacists are those involving liquids, either the propensity for liquids to be soluble in other liquids or for solids to be miscible in liquids. To begin, the first situation (liquids in liquids) will be the focus of discussion. Largely, liquid–liquid interactions involve electrostatic forces. Electrostatic forces are responsible for the existence of condensed states, such as liquids. They dictate the eventual miscibility of one liquid in another, and ultimately are the root of the organization of complex biological structures and drug–receptor interactions. Electrostatic forces cause atoms and molecules to interact, either attracting or repelling two objects.

Key Point

Ideal Gas law is $V = \dfrac{nRT}{P}$, where V = volume, n = number of moles, R = gas constant, T = temperature, and P = pressure.

Consider the liquid state of water: according to the Ideal Gas law, one gram of water at atmospheric pressure and room temperature should occupy 1358 cubic centimeters (1.358 L); i.e., if $P = 1$ atm, $n = (1$ g$)(1$ mol water/18 g water$) = 0.05555$ moles of water, $R = 0.082$ L·atm·mole^{-1}deg^{-1}, $T = 298$ K (25°C), and $V = 1.358$ L (1358 cm^3).

Yet we know this to be untrue. One gram of water under these conditions occupies approximately one cubic centimeter at room temperature. This type of deviation occurs with many liquids. Why is there such deviation from the Ideal Gas law? For water, it can be explained by understanding the strong intermolecular forces that exist between water molecules and their intramolecular origins. The presence or absence of intermolecular interactions affects not only water, but also all of the liquid substances important for pharmaceuticals. A better way to phrase the last statement is: the magnitude of intermolecular interactions affects not only water, but also all of the liquid substances important for pharmaceuticals, because intermolecular interactions always exist.

Adhesive and cohesive interactions

The fact that water is soluble in itself perhaps is not surprising, as may be the abilities of some other liquids to freely mix – or be miscible with – water. Without thinking further, the maxim 'like dissolves like' could suffice as an explanation. For example, many alcohols and water spontaneously combine to form homogeneous mixtures. But why do some liquids, such as oils, generally not mix with – or are immiscible with – water? Mixing mineral oil with water results in the separation of the two liquids, with the oil floating on top of the water. Many liquids spontaneously mix with water, while others spontaneously separate from it. The tendency for two liquids to be miscible is determined by the relative magnitude of cohesive and adhesive attractions among similar and dissimilar molecules. Cohesive interactions are those between molecules of the same kind (such as water with water). Adhesive forces are those between molecules of different kinds (such as ethanol and water). The net result of these forces, for all the involved molecules, dictates the extent to which the two liquids will interact and mix (Figure 1.1).

Cohesive forces are those between like molecules, such as water with water, ethanol with ethanol, and mineral oil with mineral oil (Figure 1.2).

Key Point

Cohesive forces are those between like molecules. Adhesive forces are those between different types of molecules.

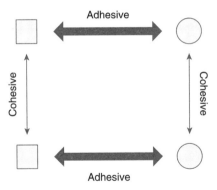

Figure 1.1 Actions of adhesive and cohesive forces

H_2O .... H_2O

$CH_3–CH_2–OH$ .... $CH_3–CH_2–OH$

Mineral oil .... Mineral oil

Figure 1.2 Examples of materials that interact via cohesive forces

Adhesive forces are those between different kinds of molecules (Figure 1.3).

$CH_3–CH_2–OH$ .... H_2O

H_2O .... Mineral oil

Figure 1.3 Examples of materials that interact via adhesive forces

If two liquids are mixed together and the sum of the cohesive forces is greater than the sum of their adhesive forces, the liquids will tend to stay in separate phases (such as oil floating on water). If the adhesive forces are stronger than the cohesive forces, the two liquids will tend to mix, to some degree. This 'degree' is a measurement known as solubility. Can solubility be predicted? The answer is yes. There are reference tables, such as Table 1.1, for many combinations to obviate the need for many calculations and provide information without needing to experiment.

When a solute dissolves in a solvent, adhesive forces have, at least to some degree, overcome cohesive forces (Figure 1.4).

Water is represented by squares, mineral oil by circles, and ethanol by triangles. In the first frame (A), the cohesive intermolecular interactions (between mineral oil molecules) are stronger than the adhesive interactions (between mineral oil and water). These liquids will be relatively insoluble in each other. In the second frame (B), adhesive intermolecular interactions (between ethanol and water) are in the same range as the cohesive interactions (ethanol–ethanol and water–water). These liquids will tend to be soluble in each other. In the third frame (C), if all three were

Table 1.1 Solubility of selected solutes		
Solute	Solvent	Solubility (g/100g)*
NaCl	Water	35.89
Glucose	Water	90.0
KCl	Water	148.0
CaCl$_2$	Water	74.5
NaCl	Glycerin	8.3
NaCl	Ethanol	0.065
KCl	Ethanol	1.88

*At standard temperature and pressure

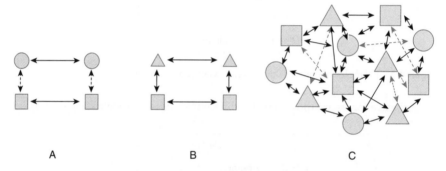

A   B   C

Figure 1.4 Illustration of solubility – adhesive forces overcoming cohesive forces

This is a conceptual illustration of cohesive and adhesive forces among three different liquids. An example of solubility using mineral oil (squares), ethanol (triangles) and water (circles). If either two, or all three, were able to dissolve in one another, this would indicate adhesive forces (solid arrows) were greater than cohesive forces (dashed lines). (A) Water and mineral oil molecules naturally attract to themselves (cohesive interactions), but not to each other (adhesive interactions), and so do not readily mix. (B) Ethanol and mineral oil have cohesive attraction, but also enough adhesive attraction that the two liquids will mix. (C) The three separate entities have some degree of solubility in each other.

capable of overcoming cohesion, the three could be soluble in one another, and the intermolecular interactions could be visualized as indicated.

Polarity

An important intermolecular property is polarity, or the tendency to form dipole moments. Recall that the dipole moment of a molecule (μ) is the net polarity, or charge separation, within the molecule, and is represented by the equation $\mu = Q \times r$, where μ is the molecule's polarity, Q is the magnitude of the charge (+ or −) at either end of the molecule, and r is the distance separating the charge centers. When the average positions of an atom's or molecule's positive and negative centers coincide, the atom or molecule is neutral, or nonpolar as illustrated in Figure 1.5.

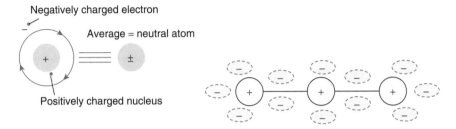

Figure 1.5 Polarity of the atom versus the molecule

(A) When considered at close range, atoms are composed of regions that differ with respect to charge. (B) The nucleus is positively charged, while electrons are negatively charged. When considered as a single entity, the atom overall is neutrally charged, with equal amounts of positive and negative charge 'cancelling' each other. Under certain conditions, most commonly when atoms are grouped and covalently bound as molecules, atoms may be ionized. More subtly, however, is the ability of molecules to form regions of charge. Though the molecule as a whole may remain neutral, if considered alone, a region may be neutral, or charged, and thus possess polar and nonpolar regions.

Key Point

An atom or molecule is polar when the average position of its electrons is asymmetrically distributed.

Polar and nonpolar molecules

Nonpolar molecules have no net dipole moment. Unless influenced by other forces, neutral molecules are incapable of substantial intermolecular interactions. Nonpolar molecules have symmetry with regard to their charge dispersion. Polar molecules have a permanent asymmetry with regard to their charge dispersion (Figure 1.6). However, nonpolar molecules can have their charge symmetry disrupted through the influences of surrounding molecules. Therefore, the key to molecular interactions is a separation of the positive and negative centers – a dipole – even if ever so briefly. Though it is relative, it should be noted that the charge that is mobile is the negative charge (electrons), and so dipole moments are the result of the movement of electrons.

Key Point

The key to molecular interactions is the separation of positive and negative centers of charge to create a dipole.

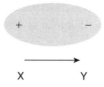

X   Y

Figure 1.6 Net dipole moment

Within this conceptual molecule are two atoms (X and Y). Y is more electronegative than X, and so electrons preferentially occupy the region around Y more than around X, creating a dipole moment.

The presence of a dipole may be a native condition of molecules, or a dipole may occur in an otherwise nonpolar molecule. The latter is fittingly called induction. A permanent dipole arises when the atoms of the molecule do not equally share the electrons of a covalently bonded molecule. This condition occurs when there are differences in electronegativity of the component atoms.

From Table 1.2, it can be observed that when comparing the electronegativities of some selected atoms from higher to lower values, we obtain F (4.1) > O (3.5) > Cl (3.0), N (3.0) > C (2.5) and H (2.2) in order of decreasing electronegativity. Recall that, moving toward the right in the Periodic Table of the Elements, atomic radii decrease, ionization energies increase, and electronegativities increase. The electronegativity of component atoms of a molecule influences the polarity of molecules. When molecules have component atoms with disparate electronegativity values, they are often polar (Figure 1.7). An exception can occur if a molecule has three-dimensional symmetry, with a net dipole moment of zero. Molecules such as hydrochloric acid have permanent dipoles and are therefore 'polar.'

Molecules of nitrogen have no difference in electronegativity, no permanent dipole, and so are considered 'nonpolar.' Why is water polar? If drawn in a linear fashion, it would appear symmetrical (H–O–H) and that it should have no net dipole moment. First, hydrogen and oxygen differ in electronegativity. This alone would dictate water should have a net dipole moment of zero though – if it were indeed linear. However, the bond angle between the two hydrogens in water molecules is 104.5°, creating nonlinear molecules. Since water molecules are not

Table 1.2 Approximate electronegativity of selected elements			
Element	Electronegativity	Element	Electronegativity
H	2.2	P	2.2
C	2.5	S	2.6
N	3.0	Cl	3.0
O	3.5	K	0.8
F	4.1	Ca	1.0
Na	0.9	Fe	1.8
Mg	1.3	I	2.5

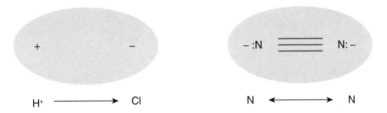

H+ ⟶ Cl   N ⟷ N

Figure 1.7 Polar elements and polar molecules

When considering molecules, as they are collections of atoms, charge can be symmetrically distributed, or it can be unbalanced. Unbalancing occurs either when two or more atoms of differing electronegativity are bonded, or it can occur when an otherwise neutral molecule has its charge induced to move to an asymmetric conformation. The charge that is actually movable is, of course, the negative charge.

linear, and there is electrostatic disparity between oxygens and hydrogens, they are able to possess a net dipole moment (Figure 1.8).

Carbon tetrachloride is also symmetrical when drawn in a linear fashion. However, in its three-dimensional conformation it truly is symmetrical, has no net dipole moment, and so is nonpolar, even though carbon and chlorine differ in electronegativity. It is the lack of an overall (net) dipole moment that causes carbon tetrachloride to be nonpolar. Nonpolar molecules do have the capacity to be polarized, perhaps briefly, by the external influences of neighboring molecules. This phenomenon is called an induced dipole, or polarization, and will be discussed below.

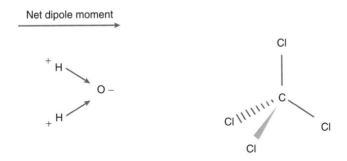

Figure 1.8 Bond angle and polarity

Since water takes on a 104.5° angle among the three atoms, a molecule that would otherwise have no net dipole moment possesses one. Carbon tetrachloride has no three-dimensional asymmetry, and so no net dipole moment.

Dipoles and polarization

All molecules are capable of forming temporary dipoles. These temporary dipoles arise because 1) electrons of a molecule are constantly in motion and 2) a given molecule is in the vicinity of other molecules. Permanent dipoles represent a difference in the average position of the centers of positive and negative charge

Table 1.3 Polarizability of selected elements	
Element	Polarizability, α (Å^3)
H	0.67
C	1.78
N	1.08
O	0.73
F	0.56
Cl	2.18
I	4.90

Polarizability, α, increases with electronegativity, and is a quantification of the relative ease an atom's (or molecule's) electrons can be distorted. The larger the value of α the more easily electrons may be distorted, and polarity induced.

within a given molecule, whereas temporary dipoles represent transient separation of positive and negative centers due to the current (transient) position of the electrons. Induction of a dipole is called polarization. Polarizability is the ease with which a distortion occurs in a molecule's charge distribution. Examples of the polarizability for some elements are shown in Table 1.3.

Key Point

Molecules can possess dipoles either permanently or temporarily.

Polarity and dipole moments

What can cause polarity? There are three variations of dipole moments between two molecules (see Figure 1.9):

A. Dipole–dipole interactions (two permanently dipole molecules; Keesom forces, ~1–7 kcal/mol). These arise from electrostatic interactions between a partially positive region of one molecule and a partially negative region of another. Some examples of molecules that form dipole–dipole interactions (D–D) include water, hydrochloric acid, alcohol, acetone, and phenol.

B. Dipole–induced dipole interactions (Debye forces, ~1–3 kcal/mol). These arise when a negative region of one molecule draws electrons in its direction from a neighboring molecule, creating a dipole on the second molecule. Some examples of molecules that form dipole-induced dipole interactions (D–I) include ethyl acetate, methylene chloride, and ether.

C. Induced dipole–induced dipole interactions (London forces, ~0.5–1 kcal/mol). These arise when one induced molecule's electron distortion induces yet another molecule to possess polarity. Some examples of molecules that form

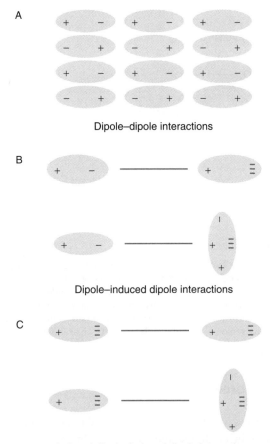

Figure 1.9 Variations of dipole moments between two molecules

(A) Dipole–dipole interactions (Keesom forces). (B) Dipole–induced dipole interactions (Debye forces). (C) Induced dipole–induced dipole interactions (London forces).

induced dipole–induced dipole interactions (I–I) include carbon disulfide, carbon tetrachloride, and hexane.

Hydrogen bonding – A special dipole–dipole interaction

Hydrogen bonding is a special example of a dipole–dipole interaction. It arises when a hydrogen atom in a polar bond attracts a nonbonding electron pair of a neighboring molecule (Figure 1.10).

Recall the requirements for hydrogen bonding. These include 1) the hydrogen must be on the positive end of a dipole (i.e., associated with more electronegative atoms, such as F, O, N), and 2) the hydrogen must be near a neighboring dipole that is highly electronegative (e.g., molecules containing F, O, N).

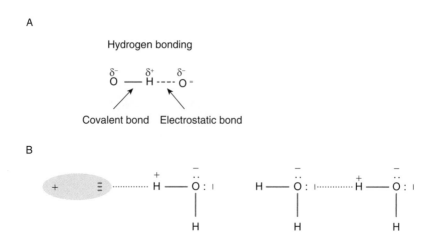

Figure 1.10 Hydrogen bonding

(A) The mechanism of the hydrogen bond. Hydrogen bonding occurs between a covalently bonded hydrogen atom and a nonbonding electron pair on a nearby molecule. Here, oxygen is more electronegative than hydrogen, leading to hydrogen bonding, a type of dipole–dipole interaction. (B) Hydrogen bonding between two molecules of water. Hydrogen bonding is a type of dipole–dipole bonding, only it involves a positively charged hydrogen portion of a molecule attracting to a negative region of a nearby molecule (left). An example is that between two molecules of water (right).

van der Waals forces

One accepted method of categorizing dipoles and polarization interactions is to include only the induced dipole–induced dipole interactions as van der Waals forces. Another method is to include all three types of interactions contributing to van der Waals forces. In either case, van der Waals forces (considered here as all three cases above) are largely responsible for the observed deviations in physical characteristics and actions that liquids display, compared with the Ideal Gas law. These deviations have broad implications for liquids in general, and begin to reveal why some liquids mix easily, while others do not. Also implied is that perhaps sometimes in exceedingly small amounts, all liquids have some degree of solubility in all others. Solubility and dissolution will be discussed in Chapter 3.

Ion–molecule interactions

In addition to van der Waals forces, actions between ions and molecules are also important when considering intermolecular interactions. Two types of inter-molecular interactions that involve ions can occur: ion–dipole and ion–induced dipole interactions. As the terms imply, these involve the actions of cations and

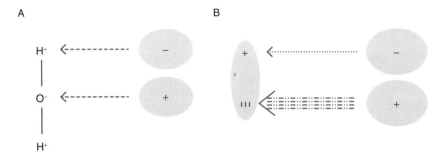

Figure 1.11 Ion–dipole and ion-induced dipole interactions

Two types of intermolecular interactions involve ions: (A) ion–dipole (close proximity of ions to a polar molecule, in this example water, left) and (B) ion–induced dipole. In each case, an ionized entity (right) interacts with areas of dipole in neighboring molecules.

anions on molecules that are either already polar (Figure 1.11A, left) or actions that cause molecules to take on dipolar character (Figure 1.11B, left).

Ion–dipoles and ion–induced dipoles are responsible for the solubility of crystals in water, where a cation is attracted to the negative center of oxygen in water (the solvent), while the anion is attracted to the positive region of the hydrogen.

Charge separation

Earlier, polarizability was defined as 'the ease with which an ion or molecule can be polarized.' To now extend this definition, 'ease' will mean 'the facility by which an electron cloud can be distorted.' As may be inferred by the discussion above, induction of dipoles in atoms or molecules simply involves affecting an electron cloud that is either evenly or unevenly distributed around an atom or molecule. This distribution can be more or less easily distorted depending on the nature (i.e., electronegativity) of the atom (or atoms comprising a molecule) and by the external pulls on the atom's (or molecule's) electron cloud from neighboring atoms or molecules. But how is 'ease' quantified? Quantifying 'ease' would allow a reasoned approach to predicting more macroscopic phenomena, such as the potential solubilities or compatibilities of liquids and solids in each other. To begin, a 'thought experiment' will be described.

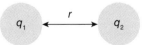

Figure 1.12 Coulomb's law relating charge and distance

Coulomb's law illustrates how the force of attraction or repulsion between two objects is related to the magnitude of charge associated with each object and the distance between the two objects.

For two charged particles, as shown in Figure 1.12, recall Coulomb's law (applied in a vacuum):

$$F = \frac{q_1 q_2}{r^2}$$

where F = the force of interaction (newtons, N), q = quantity of charge (coulombs, C) on each body, and r = distance of separation (meters, m).

Note the sign of each q is important, as, ultimately of interest is the product of both particles' charges. If q_1 and q_2 have the same charge, the product is positive, meaning the resulting force between the two will be repulsive. If they have opposite signs, the product is negative, meaning the resulting force will be attractive. Also, as the distance (r) between the two particles increases, the interaction force decreases. But, by artificially creating an electric force, nonpolar molecules can be temporarily caused to take on the characteristics of polar molecules. Now, imagine the ability to place a single molecule on an electrophoresis plate, and then create an electric field across the plate (Figure 1.13). In this situation, rather than two charged particles creating a force, two permanently separated electrodes create an electric force, which then acts on molecules between the electrodes. This imitates the effects charged molecules have on the experimental molecule.

$$\mu_{ind} = \alpha E$$

μ_{ind} = induced dipole moment (C·m²)

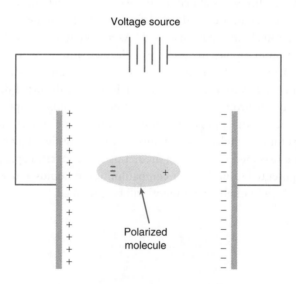

Figure 1.13 Polarization of a molecule in an electric field

Following Coulomb's law, a dipole can be temporarily induced in a molecule by placing it between two dissimilar charges (an electric field, in this case).

Table 1.4 Polarizability of selected molecules	
Molecule	**Polarizability constant, α (Å^3)**
H_2O	1.43
N_2	1.74
HCl	3.01
CH_4	2.59
HI	5.60
CCl_4	11.16

Polarizability, α, is a means of quantifying the ability of a molecule to be polarized (creation of an induced dipole) above that of the native relative polarity. The greater the value of α, the more easily the molecule can be polarized (be caused to possess a dipole). Polarizability can be used in the context of an electrophoresis field or when discussing the interactions between two molecules. α = polarizability constant = Å^3 = C·m^2/V, where C = coulombs and V = volts.

E = electrical field intensity (volts (V) or newtons/coulomb (N/C), $\simeq$ 'F' in Coulomb's law)

α = polarizability (C·m^2/V)

E is dependent on voltage and geometry (plate size, separation distance between electrodes) and is responsible for induction. The value determined by this experiment is α, the polarizability of the molecule; α is the manner by which the relative 'ease' of an atom's or molecule's electron cloud can be pulled. By creating/inducing a dipole in an otherwise nonpolar molecule, the molecule has temporarily been caused to behave as if it were polar. For now, it has been 'polarized.' The greater the polarizability of a molecule, the greater is the effect of a given electric field's intensity (induction of a dipole) on the molecule. In general, molecules with more electrons tend to have greater polarizability. Table 1.4 shows examples for the polarizability of selected molecules.

Note that 'polarizable' is not the same as 'polar' when speaking of a molecule. Both polar and nonpolar molecules can be induced. Therefore, it can be inferred that, at some point – though it may be extreme – any molecule can have a dipole induced in it, even those that already possess a dipole. This is also why it should be kept in mind that, to some degree, all liquids are soluble in all others. The obstacle is that this solubility may be so minute for two components that the practicality of creating a solution of the two is dismissible. In these cases, another pharmaceutical formulation is probably less problematic. Polarizability constants allow us to gauge, in a relative way, the potential for nonpolar molecules and other polar molecules to interact and to mix. Though Coulomb's law and a simplistic view of charge attraction and repulsion are informative, they do not completely explain 'real-life' situations.

Attraction and repulsion

Attractive and repulsive forces do not vary with distance at the same rate, as a direct interpretation of Coulomb's law would indicate. If the distance between two molecules is measured as 'r', the potential energy (PE) of attraction is proportional to r^7, whereas the PE of repulsion is proportional to r^9. So, attractive forces are 'longer range' forces than are repulsive forces. This immediately introduces a disparity from the simpler view of attractive and repulsive forces, but, as will be shown in subsequent chapters, begins to better explain observed actions of charged particles. Traditionally, when graphed, repulsive forces are positive and attractive forces are negative. Exact quantities depend on the identity of the molecules, but

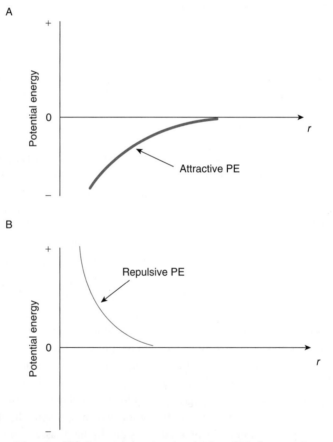

Figure 1.14 Potential energy (PE) diagrams showing the plotting of PEs for attraction and repulsion versus distance

PE between two charged molecules is inversely related to distance, as described by Coulomb's law. (A) PE of attraction (PE $\propto r^7$). (B) PE of repulsion (PE $\propto r^9$). When graphed by distance, both attractive PE (A) and repulsive PE (B) decrease with increasing distance (r). Attractive PE is traditionally assigned negative values (A), whereas repulsive PE is traditionally assigned positive values (B).

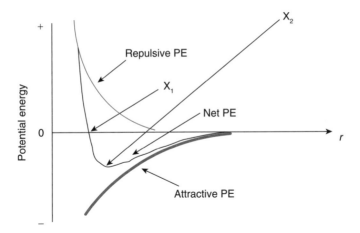

Figure 1.15 Potential energy (PE) diagram showing combined repulsive and attractive energies and the net PE

When the functions of attractive (r^7) and repulsive (r^9) PEs are combined, a net PE function (the absolute value of the difference between the attractive and repulsive plots) can also be illustrated. The net PE function indicates the existence of an overall energy 'well,' together with two points of importance for dosage form stability (X_1 and X_2).

the shape of the graph will always be consistent. If the PEs are plotted as functions of r, the result are the graphs as illustrated in Figure 1.14.

When the two PE plots are superimposed (Figure 1.15), the difference between the two functions (r^7 and r^9 for attraction and repulsion, respectively) becomes more apparent. As these functions are combined, the net PE results in the net plot as illustrated.

The attractive forces are van der Waals forces, while the repulsive forces are electrostatic. It can be seen that attractive potential is predominant at a longer range than is repulsive potential. That is, van der Waals forces are exerted over a more protracted range than are electrostatic forces. This means that molecules tend to be drawn toward each other until a certain distance, X_1 (Figure 1.15), is approached, where repulsive and attractive forces are at equilibrium. If molecules move more closely than X_1 the repulsive PE increases rapidly and becomes the dominant force. The point where the attractive and repulsive forces balance (the x-intercept closest to the y-axis) is the collision diameter, X_1. X_2, the outer PE minimum, represents an 'optimum' distance two molecules will tend to assume, where the attractive and repulsive forces balance. X_2 is the most energetically favorable distance between two molecules. However, closer than this point the electron clouds of molecules would interpenetrate. At distances (r) beyond the PE minimum X_2, the net PE again reaches a value approximately that of X_1. Further reaches of the PE plot will be illustrated later; the outer values will have importance when considering stability issues of disperse systems.

Why are the deviations from Coulomb's law important? When considering the force of attraction (F_{att}) between two molecules:

- For dipole–dipole interactions, both molecules already possess a charge and Coulomb's law becomes $F_{att} \propto (\mu_1\mu_2/r^7)$, where magnitude of the dipole in the molecules, μ, is a major factor.
- For dipole–induced dipole interactions, the major factor for the dipolar molecule is still μ, while the major factor for the induced molecule is α, its polarizability constant. Therefore, for dipole–induced dipole interactions, $F_{att} \propto (\mu_1\alpha_2/r^7)$.
- For induced dipole–induced dipole interactions $F_{att} \propto (\alpha_1\alpha_2/r^7)$. This last variation can be envisioned as the attractive force existing between two molecules in a pure nonpolar liquid. In this case, since both molecules are identical, $\alpha_1 = \alpha_2$, $F_{att} \propto (\alpha^2/r^7)$.

If considering attractive forces in a pure polar liquid, all three types of forces are possible among molecules, and so have to be included, so $F_{att} \alpha (\mu^2 + \mu\alpha + \alpha^2/r^7)$, comprising μ^2 of dipole–dipole interactions, $\mu\alpha$ of dipole–induced dipole interactions and α^2 of induced dipole–induced dipole interactions occurring in the liquid.

Intermolecular interactions

What factors influence the development of molecular interactions in liquids? From the discussion, it can be said μ, α and r are the greatest influences. The larger the dipole moment (μ), the greater the attractive force. The larger the polarizability (α), the greater the attractive force, and the greater the distance between interacting molecules (r), the smaller the attractive force. There is one other common variable that can influence intermolecular interactions. This is temperature. As temperature increases, molecules are supplied with more kinetic energy, their movement increases, thereby decreasing the opportunities for the three types of interactions to occur, as well as supplying energy to overcome any of the discussed intermolecular interactions, if they do occur. When a liquid is heated, its density decreases, meaning there is more distance between molecules. The effects of temperature on liquids will be discussed further in Chapter 3. For now, it is important to keep in mind that temperature has important effects on intermolecular interactions.

How about intermolecular interactions between solids and liquids? Some of the same principles that are important for liquid–liquid interactions apply to liquid–solid interactions. However, in order to completely address solid–liquid interactions, dissolution and solubility need to be discussed. These are distinct topics and will be addressed in Chapter 3.

Summary

In summary, the composition of a liquid dictates its physical characteristics. The difference in composition between two or more liquids in contact with each other dictates their propensity to mix. Within a single liquid, and within a mixture of liquids, act three important intermolecular interactions. These are dipole–dipole, dipole–induced dipole, and induced dipole–induced dipole interactions. With ion-containing liquids, ion–dipole and ion–induced dipole interaction are also possible. At a molecular level, this provides an insight into why some liquids will mix together, while others will not – at least to a useful extent. In addition, since these interactions require favorable molecular orientations, increasing temperature decreases the propensity of molecules in a liquid to be able to form intermolecular interactions, and so to interact in a meaningful way at macromolecular level.

Self-assessment questions

1. Why do liquids not obey the Ideal Gas law with regard to the volumes the liquids occupy?

2. In order for two liquids to be miscible, which forces should be greater than which?

3. What is the fundamental origin of intermolecular interactions?

4. Which type of intermolecular interaction is only dependent on a liquid's polarizability constant (α)?

5. Describe and differentiate the three main intermolecular interactions that pertain to pure liquids.

6. Within the context of the current discussion, differentiate between attractive and repulsive forces that act between molecules.

7. Explain the difference between adhesive and cohesive forces.

8. Explain polarity and polarizability pertaining to molecules. Explain how knowing a liquid's polarizability could be helpful when choosing another liquid that will be compatible.

9. List different types of dipole moments for molecules. How can understanding a liquid's dipole moment be useful when considering liquid–liquid miscibility and preparation of drug delivery systems?

10. Speculate when and why it might be desirable to keep charged drug delivery system molecules at distances further apart than the net PE minimum for the system.

2

Pharmaceutical solvents

Learning objectives

Upon completion of this chapter, you should be able to answer the following questions:

- What is a solvent? What do solvents do?
- What are the differences among polar, semipolar, and nonpolar solvents?
- Define what a dielectric constant is.
- What is the significance of a solvent's dielectric constant?
- What are the functions of pharmaceutical solvents?

What is a solvent?

Solvents are very important components in pharmaceuticals, enabling the delivery of liquid drugs that otherwise might require a solid or powder form of delivery to patients. They also can impart palatability to oral delivery systems and act as the delivery vehicle for many drugs. There are many solvents available that could solvate drugs and pharmaceutically-related materials, but many cannot be considered for use in drug delivery systems because of their toxicity, volatility, instability, and/or flammability. Thus, despite many solvents' attractive chemical attributes, the need for patient safety narrows the number of candidates that are of practical use in drug delivery systems. Some solvents can be used topically, but are not acceptable for internal use. A solvent is (usually) a liquid capable of dissolving another substance, resulting in a solution. However, in practice, the term 'solvent' is also often applied to a liquid that suspends a dispersed solid or liquid without true dissolution occurring. Solutions, which will be more thoroughly discussed in Chapter 3, are composed of two components: a solvent and a solute. A solute is the component that is being dissolved to create a solution. Again, in practice, the solute can be meant to be the substance that is dispersed, but this is not a technically accurate application of the term 'solute.' The act of dissolving a solute in a solvent is solvation. Whichever component's physical state is preserved when a solution is formed is considered the solvent in the system. An elementary example is the combination of sodium chloride, a solid, with liquid water. Unless the sodium chloride is present in large excess, the resulting combination results in a liquid, and it can be inferred that water is the solvent in this system and sodium chloride is the solute because the liquid is the preserved state.

NaCl (solid) + H_2O (liquid) = Liquid
Solute   Solvent

The qualifying statement leads to the following extended definition: 'If all components are in the same physical state, the component present in the greatest proportion is considered the solvent for the system.' For example, ethanol can dissolve in water or water can dissolve in ethanol. The identification of which component is the solvent depends on the relative weights (not usually volumes for alcoholic solutions) of each. If the amount of water is greater than that of ethanol, water is considered the solvent and ethanol the solute. If ethanol is present in a greater amount than that of water the converse will be true. The extent to which a solute can dissolve in a solvent is its solubility in that particular solvent. The extent and rate of solution are two different concepts, but can be related.

Solubility and dissolution rate will be discussed in Chapter 3. At this point, the variety of solvents available, and their different means of interacting with solutes, are important to understand. Generally, most solvents used in drug delivery systems are polar. Therefore, as described in Chapter 1, most of our solvents function using repulsive and attractive intermolecular interactions – van der Waals forces (which in this text include all three of the forces, dipole–dipole, dipole–induced dipole, and induced dipole–induced dipole) – as well as ion–dipole, ion–induced dipole, and electrostatic repulsive forces (see Chapter 1). Solvent actions occur as a result of repulsive and attractive forces at work, which produces a solution. Solutions will be further discussed in Chapter 3.

Utility of solvents

Why are solvents useful as part of drug delivery systems? Obviously, dissolution of drugs and other components of drug delivery systems is a primary physical pharmacy function. In addition, if a liquid delivery system is desired, the proper solvent must be used. Solvents also can influence palatability of oral systems and improve (or weaken) product stability. However, since many drugs need to be delivered in solution, the choice of solvent is often tantamount to creating successful delivery systems.

Types of solvents

In Chapter 1 it was emphasized that presence or absence of a dipole (polarity) is an important property for substances because it dictates much of the intermolecular interaction that occurs among molecules. Therefore, it should not be surprising that solvents can be categorized based on this property. Solvents comprise three types: polar, semipolar, and nonpolar. When selecting the best solvent for a drug delivery system, a solvent from the appropriate category that best matches the property of the solute (the material being solvated) is chosen, as much as is practical.

Key Point

Solvents comprise three types: polar, semipolar, and nonpolar.

Polar solvents

Some solutes ionize when in aqueous solution, while others do not. Some are lipophilic, some hydrophilic. Polar solvents are strong dipolar molecules that often employ hydrogen bonding as an interaction type. Polar solvents also sometimes act by breaking covalent bonds of a solute, causing solute ionization. Polar solvents, including among others, water and alcohols, are the most prominent solvents used in drug delivery systems. The most common alcohols used as solvents include ethanol, isopropyl alcohol, glycerin, and propylene glycol. Again, some of these are useful for external applications but may be useful for internal applications only in small amounts, if at all, due to toxicity problems. Common solutes for which polar solvents are used include other polar solvents (such as alcohols, aldehydes, and ketones), sugars, and other compounds with –OH groups. Polar solvents typically have dielectric constants greater than 50 (Figure 2.1).

Key Point

Polar solvents are those whose dielectric constants are 50 and greater.

Semipolar solvents

Semipolar solvents typically are strong dipolar molecules that do not form hydrogen bonds but can induce polarity in nonpolar molecules (D–I and I–I; see Chapter 1) – both solutes and solvents. Solvents are considered 'semipolar' when their dielectric constants are between 20 and 50. When used for induction of a nonpolar solvent, such as benzene, the semipolar solvent is acting as an intermediate solvent. An example of this is when acetone ($\varepsilon \sim 21$) increases the solubility of ether ($\varepsilon \sim 4$) in water ($\varepsilon \sim 80$). Semipolar solvents include acetone, aldehydes and other ketones, some esters, and nitro-compounds (Figure 2.2).

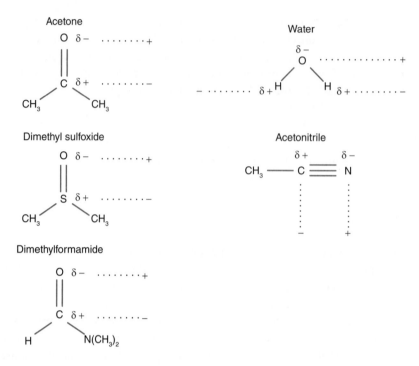

Figure 2.1 Actions of polar solvents

Polar solvents are those whose dielectric constants are 50 and greater. Polar solvents utilize permanent dipole moments and hydrogen bonding to enable interaction with electron-rich regions of solutes.

Key Point

Semipolar solvents are those whose dielectric constants are between 20 and 50.

Nonpolar solvents

Nonpolar solvents possess little or no dipolar character. Although they tend to be unable to independently form dipoles (i.e., depend on induced dipoles) they can utilize induced dipole–induced dipole (ID–ID) interactions for dissolving appropriate solutes. Nonpolar solvents have dielectric constants between 1 and 20, and include fixed oils, carbon tetrachloride, and chloroform among others (Figure 2.3). Ionic and polar solutes have little-to-no solubility in nonpolar solvents. However, oils, fats, and fatty acids dissolve well in nonpolar solvents.

Key Point

Nonpolar solvents are those whose dielectric constants are between 1 and 20.

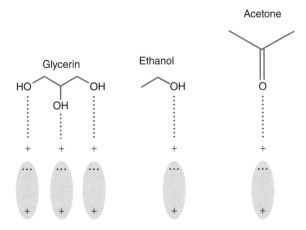

Figure 2.2 Semipolar solvents and induced polarity

Common semipolar solvents, with dielectric constants, include ethanol (25), glycerin (46), and acetone (21). Semipolar solvents are not as polar as solvents like water but can still induce dipoles in other molecules, solvents, or solutes.

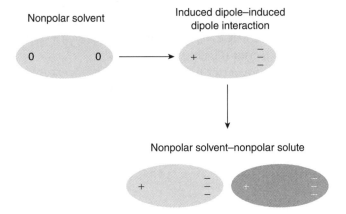

Figure 2.3 Actions of nonpolar solvents

Nonpolar solvents act mainly through induced dipole–induced dipole interactions with other solvents and solutes.

The dielectric constant

An objective method for matching solvents and solutes is to utilize their dielectric constants (ε) to determine, on a 'spectrum,' how polar or nonpolar substances are. The dielectric constant is a relative measure, for a substance, of how much electrostatic energy can be stored per unit volume of material when a unit of voltage is applied; it is quantified as the ratio of the capacitance in a chamber containing the material to that when only a vacuum exits in the chamber:

$$C = \frac{q}{V}$$

where C = capacitance (farads), q = charge (coulombs/volts), and V = volts between plates.

$$\epsilon = \frac{C_x}{C_0}$$

where C_x is the capacitance of the material in question (our potential solvent or solute) and C_0 is the capacitance of a reference material. Usually the 'reference material' is a vacuum and so C_0 is the capacitance measured in a vacuum, and is traditionally assigned a value of one. Since ϵ is a ratio, it does not have units.

Aside from providing a means of matching solvents and solutes, the dielectric constant measures the ability of a solvent to reduce the attractive forces holding solute molecules together. The dielectric constant is sometimes referred to as permittivity. For pharmaceutical applications, the dielectric constant measures how easily two oppositely charged ions or molecules may be separated when a specific substance acts as the medium. An example of this application is a prediction of how well a solvent will be able to separate the ions composing a crystalline structure, such as sodium chloride (Figure 2.4).

The more polar the solvent (the higher/larger ϵ is), the more easily that solvent can overcome attractive forces within the crystal or other innate stabilizing forces

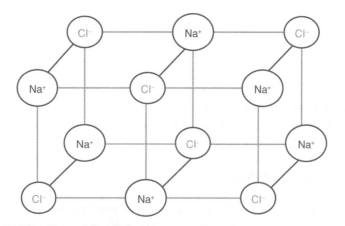

Figure 2.4   Crystalline structure of sodium chloride

Sodium chloride is arranged in octahedral geometry, composed of ionic bonds. In order to dissolve sodium chloride, the relative pull of these ionic bonds must be overcome. The dielectric constants differ greatly for the two materials (NaCl = 6.1; H_2O = 80.4), which contributes to propensity of sodium chloride to dissolve in water.

that may exist, and separate the components (ions in the case of sodium chloride). A larger value for ε implies easier solute separation and a more polar solvent. Polar solvents have large dielectric constants, nonpolar solvents have small dielectric constants, and semipolar solvents have intermediate dielectric constants. Some measured dielectric constants are shown in Table 2.1.

When considering dielectric constants of potential solvents for a drug delivery system, it should be remembered that liquids with low dielectric constants are very weak at separating charges – so weak that interactions between solute ions can actually be improved if dispersed in such liquids – an indication that the opposite of stabilization and separation of ions is occurring.

Classification of solvent types based on their dielectric constants is shown in Table 2.2.

Polar solvents are those with dielectric constants greater than 50. Water ($\varepsilon = 80.4$) is a polar solvent capable of overcoming the attractive force between crystal

Table 2.1 Examples of dielectric constants of some materials	
Material	**Dielectric constant, ε***
N-Methylformamide	182.0
Formamide	110.0
Hydrogen cyanide	95.4
Hydrogen peroxide	84.2
Water	80.4
Hydrazine	52.9
Glycerin	47.0
Methanol	32.6
Ethanol	24.3
Acetone	20.7
Isopropyl alcohol	18.3
Calcium fluoride	7.4
Acetic acid	6.2
Sodium chloride	6.1
Chloroform	4.8
Potassium chloride	4.6
Diethyl ether	4.3
Hydrochloric acid	4.1
Olive oil	3.1
Mannitol	3.0
Benzene	2.3
Pentane	1.8
Air	1.0

*ε units are farads/meter = F/m; also denoted permittivity.

Table 2.2 Solvent categorization based on dielectric constant	
Dielectric constant, ε	Solvent type
1–20	Nonpolar
20–50	Semipolar
>50	Polar

ions by a factor of nearly 80 compared to the reference (vacuum, reference = 1) (Figure 2.5).

Polar solvents (such as water, ε = 80.4) dissolve ionic solutes and polar substances, whereas nonpolar solvents (e.g., pentane, ε = 1.8) cannot appreciably do so. However, pentane can dissolve nonpolar substances like oils and fats (Figure 2.6). Common semipolar solvents include those with mid-range ε values, such as acetone (ε = 20.7, Figure 2.7). Also, semipolar solvents can sometimes be combined with either polar or nonpolar solvents to improve solubility of a third component. For example, acetone (ε = 20.7) increases the solubility of diethyl ether (ε = 4.3) in water (ε = 80.4). Acetone, in this situation, is then referred to as a cosolvent.

Cosolvents are solvents used in conjunction with primary solvents. Cosolvents are used to increase drug solubility. They are usually water-miscible organic

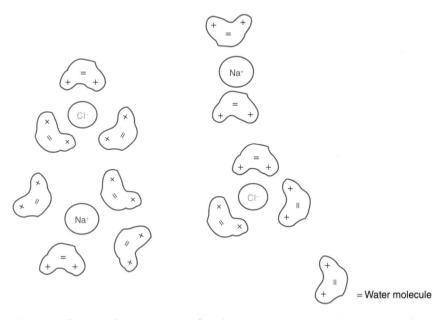

Figure 2.5 Conceptual representation of a polar solvent (water) overcoming the attractive force between Na⁺ and Cl⁻. Water, a polar solvent, can effectively overcome the attractive forces of many ionizable crystals, such as sodium chloride, and separate and solvate the ions.

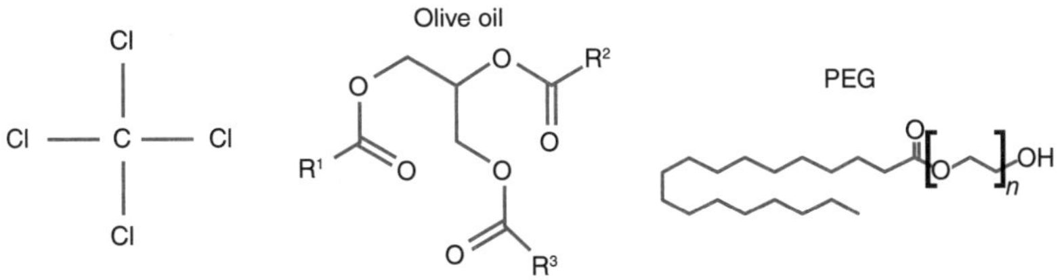

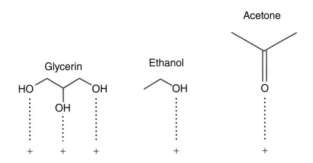

Figure 2.6 Nonpolar solvent actions on nonpolar solutes

Common nonpolar solvents, with dielectric constants, include carbon tetrachloride (2.2), olive oil (3.1), and polyethylene glycol (PEG) 400 (12.4).

Figure 2.7 Actions of semipolar solvents

Common semipolar solvents with dielectric constants, include glycerin (47.0), ethanol (24.3), and acetone (20.7).

solvents, meaning they are organic in nature, but have a reasonable degree of solubility in water. Addition of a solvent with lower polarity (lower dielectric constant) than water makes the combined 'solvent' less water-like, improving solubility of drugs with less polar nature. Two examples of liquids commonly used as cosolvents are ethanol and glycerin.

Some situations where considering the dielectric constant of a solvent might be helpful are illustrated below:

1. If there is a need for mixing two solvents for a system (i.e., using a solvent and a cosolvent), the weighted average of the individual dielectric values approximates the resultant true dielectric constant of the mixture. This situation can occur if it is known that a drug is not stable in water alone, but an aqueous-based delivery system is needed. In this situation, water-miscible solvents (like ethanol, a polyethylene glycol (PEG), or glycerin) may be useful as either the initial drug solvent or as a cosolvent because ethanol and PEG are semipolar, complementing the polar solvent, water. An example appears below:

If a 30% ethanol in water preparation is required for a drug delivery system, and references state $\varepsilon_{ethanol} = 24.3$ F/m and the $\varepsilon_{water} = 80.4$ F/m, an estimate of the mixed ε can be made as a weighted average, as follows:

$$0.30(\varepsilon_{ethanol}) + 0.70(\varepsilon_{water}) = 0.30(24.3 \text{ F/m}) + 0.70(80.4 \text{ F/m})$$
$$= 7.3 + 56.3 = 63.6 \text{ F/m}.$$

If the measured ε for this mixture is 59.5, the estimate may be close enough for this application. This estimation method may be accurate enough for some applications, though it cannot be used for mixed solvents when considering non-electrolytes.

2. Solubilities of solutes in different solvents possessing similar dielectric constants are similar. Therefore, potential solubility of a solute can be estimated by comparing solvents with similar dielectric constants.

If a 60% (w/w) ethanol ($\varepsilon = 24.3$) in water ($\varepsilon = 80.4$) mixture is needed for a particular preparation, and then sodium chloride is to be added to the resulting mixture, can an estimate of sodium chloride solubility be made without knowing its true solubility in the 60% solvent solution? The answer sometimes is yes. Again, estimating the resulting dielectric constant ε:

$$0.60(24.3) + 0.40(80.4) = 46.7.$$

Glycerin has a dielectric constant (47.0) similar to the 60% hydroalcoholic solution. If the solubility of sodium chloride in glycerin can be found (and it can, and is 8.3 g/100 g glycerin), the estimate can sometimes be used. The true solubility of sodium chloride in 60% (w/w) ethanol in water is 6.3 g/100 g. The estimate may be close enough, depending on the application of the preparation. It should be noted that the estimate would be closer to true solubility if percent by volume, rather than by weight were used.

Summary

In summary, solvents are central to many aspects that dictate the ultimate actions of drug delivery systems. Solutes dissolve in specific solvents and to varying degrees, depending on the solvent. Ultimately, dissolution leads to a solution, the most basic liquid dosage form – aside from pure liquids.

Solvents can be categorized based on their polarity, as polar, semipolar, and nonpolar solvents. Each type of solvent will be most useful when dissolving solutes that possess similar polarity characteristics to that of the solvent. A means of evaluating and predicting the ability of a solvent to dissolve a solute is the use of dielectric constants. Matching dielectric constants of substances usually provides optimum dissolution, as solute and solvent polarity are matched. If a good match is not available, sometimes a cosolvent can be used to provide improved dissolution of a solute.

Choice of the proper solvent is tantamount to providing the best solutions. Solutions are sometimes the end-product and sometimes an intermediate or component of the final drug delivery system.

Self-assessment questions

1. What is a solvent?

2. Without knowing the dielectric constant for potassium chloride, which would you expect to be the best solvent for potassium chloride – water, acetone, or olive oil?

3. Provided the dielectric constant for potassium chloride ($\varepsilon = 4.6$), which would you expect to be the better solvent for potassium chloride – water ($\varepsilon = 80.4$) or acetone ($\varepsilon = 20.7$)?

4. List the three types of solvents discussed and differentiate them from one another. Describe how and why each type of solvent would, or would not 'work' for dissolving various solutes (e.g., polar, nonpolar, hydrophilic, hydrophobic).

5. What is a dielectric constant for a substance?

6. How can knowing the dielectric constant of a substance be helpful when selecting a solvent or solute for a drug delivery system?

7. If the dielectric constant of calcium sulfate is 5.6 F/m and that of glycerin is 47.0 F/m, would you predict glycerin would be an effective solvent for calcium sulfate?

8. If a 10% glycerin-in-water preparation is required for a drug delivery system, and references state $\varepsilon_{glycerin} = 47.0$ F/m and the $\varepsilon_{water} = 80.4$ F/m, what is the estimated resulting dielectric constant of the solution?

9. What are the functions of pharmaceutical solvents?

10. What category would best fit the solvent mixture in question 8 – polar, semi-polar, or nonpolar?

3

Solubility and dissolution

Learning objectives

Upon completion of this chapter, you should be able to answer the following questions:

- What is a solution?
- What is the difference between solubility and dissolution?
- What variables control a solute's solubility?
- What variables control dissolution?
- What do solubility and dissolution have to do with each other?

Solubility, dissolution, and dissolution rate

Solubility and dissolution are different concepts, but are related. Solubility is the capacity of a solute to dissolve in a pure solvent. This means the maximum amount of solute that the pure solvent can hold in solution, at specified environmental conditions. Beyond this saturation concentration, a solute cannot further dissolve in the amount of solvent provided. It can exist tenuously in a supersaturated condition, but will eventually revert to the solvent's true capacity. But what occurs between solutes and solvents that bestows the variability observed in solubilities in a given solvent? Solubility is a thermodynamic process: the system will tend to arrive at a point of lowest potential energy (PE) (Gibbs free energy), which is most thermodynamically stable. When we speak of solubility, it is understood to mean the ultimate outcome, without regard to how fast it occurs. Solubility provides us with important information, but it only tells us the endpoint, not how long it takes to get there.

Solutes vary not only in the extent to which they will dissolve, but also how quickly they will reach their respective solubility limits. Solubility and dissolution rate are two distinct phenomena. Dissolution rate is a kinetic process. A solute may have poor solubility in a solvent, yet its dissolution rate may be rapid. Conversely, a solute can be very soluble, yet require a protracted amount of time to arrive at the final, saturation concentration. Some solutes dissolve very rapidly in appropriate solvents, while others can take an inordinate amount of time to reach a desired concentration, or saturation. Why is this?

What affects total solubility, without regard for the time it takes to reach it? The answer is there are many parameters affecting solubility, which make it impossible to explain in a single statement or equation.

Solubility

Solubility can be expressed in precise or general terms. General terms include such categorizations as 'slightly soluble,' 'soluble,' 'insoluble.' Precise terms are expressed with units such as 'g/L,' 'g/100 g,' 'g%,' or 'mg/mL.' In either case, the object is to provide a measure of how much solute will ultimately dissolve in a given quantity of solvent – a capacity. It is the resting point for the equilibrium between undissolved solute and solubilized solute. As discussed in Chapters 1 and 2, the propensity for a solute to dissolve in a solvent is fundamentally dependent on intermolecular interactions, which lead to cohesive and adhesive forces between similar and dissimilar molecules. The extent to which cohesive and adhesive forces prevail correlates with the capacity a solvent has for a solute. This capacity will often also be dependent on specified conditions of temperature and atmospheric pressure, as solubility usually varies with changes in these two parameters. Once the capacity of a solvent to dissolve any further solute is reached, further addition of solute will simply result in settling of the solute to the bottom of the container (when considering aqueous-based solutions). Solutions can be made that are supersaturated by altering the temperature at which the solvent is added, and a concentration over the natural capacity at unaltered temperature of the solvent can be achieved. However, supersaturated solutions are unstable and easily precipitate out excess solute to reach the solubility capacity at the given temperature.

The dissolution rate can be expressed via the Noyes–Whitney equation:

$$\frac{dm}{dt} = A\frac{D}{d}(C_s - C_b)$$

where

dm/dt = solute dissolution rate (kg·s^{-1})

m = mass of dissolved material (kg)

t = time (s)

A = surface area of the solute particle (m^2)

D = diffusion coefficient (m·s^{-1}), which is related, in part, to the viscosity of the solvent, and will be discussed further below.

d = thickness of the concentration gradient (m)

C_s = particle surface (saturation) concentration (kg or moles/L)

C_b = concentration in the bulk solvent/solution (kg or moles/L).

Key Point

Solubility is an endpoint representing dissolution capacity. Dissolution rate can be expressed using the Noyes–Whitney equation.

In this model, C_s is the saturation concentration of the solute in question in the given solvent. The intrinsic dissolution rate ($kg \cdot m^{-2} \cdot s$) is the dissolution rate of a pure solute, normalized to the solute surface area, and actually decreases with time. The Noyes–Whitney equation is illustrated in Figure 3.1.

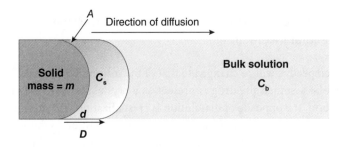

Figure 3.1 Noyes–Whitney parameters for dissolution rate

Dissolution (with rate dm/dt) occurs from a solid with mass = m and surface area = A, from the saturation concentration at the particle surface (C_s) to the concentration in the bulk solution (C_b). Concentration follows a gradient d with a coefficient D.

The Noyes–Whitney equation provides much practical information relevant to the dissolution process. When we look at the equation parameters, we see the equation predicts the following:

- The diffusion coefficient, D, which is in part related to solvent viscosity, will decrease with increasing solvent viscosity, and decreasing dissolution rate, dm/dt. That is, D is inversely proportional to viscosity; D will be discussed shortly.
- Dissolution rate (dm/dt) will be faster with smaller particles because surface area (A) increases as particle size decreases. So, trituration or micronization of particles will usually speed up dissolution.
- Some type of stirring or agitation during dissolution will decrease the diffusion gradient (d) by removing solute molecules more quickly from the particle surface, increasing dissolution rate, dm/dt.

- If the solute is ionizable and/or a weak electrolyte, altering the solvent pH can affect the surface/saturation concentration, C_s. Depending on the characteristics of the solute and solvent, this change could either increase or decrease C_s, either decreasing or increasing the concentration gradient, respectively, and increase or decrease dissolution rate, respectively.

Solubility is a key point, representing capacity. Dissolution rate can be expressed using the Noyes–Whitney equation.

Parameters that affect total solubility

I. The nature and strength of solute–solvent attractions (intermolecular interactions)
II. Polarities of the solute and solvent
III. The thermodynamics of the dissolution
IV. Temperature
V. Ionization of solute and solvent, and pH of the solvent

I. The nature and strength of solute–solvent attractions (intermolecular interactions)

First, the perspective will be changed to that of the solvent. For the sake of discussion, it will be assumed the drug is present as a crystalline structure. Therefore, for this section, the opposite of dissolution is crystallization. The attraction of the solvent for solute molecules (adhesive forces) is in opposition to the attraction of solute molecules to themselves (cohesive forces), and these opposing actions can be represented using an equilibrium equation (Figure 3.2).

$$\text{Solute + Solvent} \underset{\text{crystallization}}{\overset{\text{dissolution}}{\rightleftharpoons}} \text{Solution}$$

Figure 3.2   Dissolution equilibrium

If the solvent sufficiently interacts with solvent particles, the solute intermingles with the solvent. The crystalline structure of the solute is reduced and separated by the solvent into individual ions, atoms or molecules. This process can be visualized in Figure 3.3.

Key Point

Dissolution is a thermodynamically favorable process. In order for a solute to dissolve in a solvent, the process must be thermodynamically favorable.

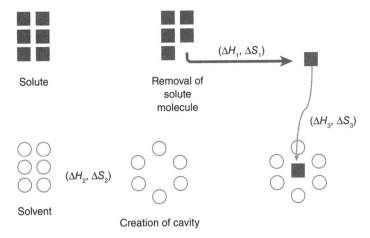

Figure 3.3 Conceptual visualization of dissolution

The dissolution process can be viewed as three thermodynamic steps: 1) creation of an opening (cavity) within solvent molecules with the Gibbs free energy change of ΔH_1 and entropy change of ΔS_1; 2) removal of a solute molecule from a particle (ΔH_2, ΔS_2); and 3) insertion of the particle into the solvent cavity (ΔH_3, ΔS_3).

In the initial step, the solute is removed (attracted away from) its crystal. Following this, a space is created in a group of solvent molecules and the isolated solute molecule is inserted into this space. Since the solute molecules open to create a space for the solute molecule, the size or surface area of the solute molecule is important. Solute molecules must contact the solute, so large solute molecules will have a smaller surface area for solvent contact than will smaller molecules when considered as a whole. Therefore, solubility tends to decrease with increasing molecular surface area.

II. Polarities of the solute and solvent

The influences of polarity of the solute and solvent were discussed in Chapter 1 in terms of molecular dipoles – innate or induced. If the solvent contains polar molecules (e.g., water), polar solutes will be more attracted to the solvent than will nonpolar solutes. Nonpolar solutes will have some attraction to polar molecules, via dipole–induced dipole actions, but the magnitudes of these attractions will be much smaller. Therefore, polar solutes will generally be more soluble in polar solvents.

III. The thermodynamics of the dissolution

Recall the Gibbs free energy equation, $\Delta G = \Delta H - T\Delta S$, where ΔG is the change in Gibbs free energy (energy to do work), ΔH is the change in enthalpy, and ΔS is the change in entropy. Increases in enthalpy are thermodynamically unfavorable when taken alone, whereas increases in entropy are favorable when taken alone. Overall, to be thermodynamically favorable, a negative ΔG is required. This equation can be used to represent the three steps of dissolution described above, keeping the system isothermal.

Using Figure 3.3, step one of the dissolution scheme, breaking of the solute lattice to free a solute particle, can be represented with ΔH_1 and ΔS_1. This action increases enthalpy but decreases entropy ($\Delta H \uparrow, \Delta S \downarrow$).

Step two, the opening of the solvent, can be represented with ΔH_2 and ΔS_2. This action increases enthalpy (ΔH), while the change in entropy depends on whether or not the solvent molecules need to be ordered to allow the solute molecule in ($\Delta H \uparrow, \Delta S \uparrow\downarrow$).

Step three, the insertion of solute into the solvent, can be represented with ΔH_3 and ΔS_3. This action increases enthalpy but decreases entropy ($\Delta H \uparrow, \Delta S \downarrow$).

Overall, the process involves enthalpy (H) changes of ΔH_1, ΔH_2 and ΔH_3. It also involves entropy (S) changes of ΔS_1, ΔS_2 and ΔS_3. Thermodynamically, we are interested in the total, final change only. For the three-step process, the free energy of solution is: $\Delta G_{soln} = (\Delta H_1 + \Delta H_2 + \Delta H_3) - T(\Delta S_1 + \Delta S_2 + \Delta S_3)$. As stated above, in order for a solute to dissolve, the overall ΔG must be negative. This obviously is the case when $\Sigma\Delta H$ is less than $\Sigma\Delta S$ ($\Sigma\Delta H < \Sigma\Delta S$), regardless of the individual values.

Another way of looking at this three-step process is simply considering the sum of work done to accomplish each of the steps. If solvent molecules are labeled as '1', and solute molecules as '2', the simple 'work equations' are: 1) step one gains PE and the work done $= w_{22}$ (work of two solute molecules); the work in step two $= w_{11}$; the increase in PE, or work, is $-w_{12}$ for closing the hole, and an additional $-w_{12}$ for net work in the final step. Therefore, the overall work $= w_{22} + w_{11} - 2w_{12}$. Using either approach, the three-step dissolution process must be thermodynamically favorable in order for it to occur. That said, even a thermodynamically favorable change only can occur – there is no certainty it will occur.

IV. Temperature

Temperature affects solubility and is also thermodynamically related. The effect of temperature on solubility depends whether the particular dissolution process is endothermic or exothermic in nature and the ambient environmental conditions. Endothermic processes are reactions in which heat is absorbed ($\Delta H > 0$). Exothermic processes are those in which heat is released ($\Delta H < 0$). If the ambient temperature is relatively high, exothermic dissolution processes will be inhibited, while endothermic dissolution processes will be improved. So, high ambient temperatures will increase the solubility of solutes with endothermic dissolution processes, but decrease the solubility of those with exothermic processes.

V. Ionization of solute and solvent, and pH of the solvent

It is assumed the reader is familiar with the Henderson–Hasselbalch equation, $pH = pK_a + \log([A^-]/[HA])$, where $[A^-]$ = molar concentration of a conjugate base (ionized form), and $[HA]$ = molar concentration of an undissociated (unionized) weak acid. The pH of the solvent can greatly impact the solubility of ionizable solutes. Acidic drugs are less soluble in acid solutions because more of the drug tends to be in the unionized form, which is less able to interact with the solvent (water) than the ionized form. The dependence of the solubility of an acidic drug on ionization of the drug, in acidic conditions, is represented by equation A:

$$pH - pK_a = \log\left(\frac{S - S_0}{S_0}\right)$$

where S is the solubility of the of the ionized drug and S_0 is the solubility of the unionized drug.

The solubility of basic drugs in relation to pH is represented by equation B:

$$pH - pK_a = \log\left(\frac{S_0}{S - S_0}\right)$$

where S is the solubility of the of the unionized drug and S_0 is the solubility of the ionized drug.

The zwitterion form has the lowest solubility, S_0. At pH values below the isoelectric point (pK_a), equation B is used. For pH values above the isoelectric point, equation A is used.

The previous discussion tells us why there are specific solubility limits, but not why there are different dissolution rates.

Dissolution

What is dissolution, exactly? In simple terms it is the process of a solute dispersing/dissociating in a solvent, forming a molecular-level, chemically and physically homogenous dispersion, called a solution. In contrast to solubility, when we speak of dissolution, it is understood that rate is a major consideration. Solubility is an endpoint. Dissolution is a process. There are different types of solutions of course. Examples of solutions, with all phase combinations, are shown in Table 3.1.

For this text, discussion is focused on liquid-in-liquid and solid-in-liquid solutions – and so the solubility and dissolution for such solutions. Within 'solid-in-liquid solutions,' there are two major types of dissolution. In the first type, the solution's phase contains the same solute chemical entity as is found in the original solid phase. Upon removal of solvent, the solute can be recovered unaltered by the dissolution process. An example is the dissolution of sucrose in water (Figure 3.4).

Table 3.1	Examples of different types of solutions	
Solute	Solvent	Example
Gas	Gas	Air
Liquid	Gas	Water vapor in air
Solid	Gas	Iodine vapor in air
Gas	Liquid	Carbonated water
Liquid	Liquid	Alcohol in water
Solid	Liquid	Sucrose in water
Gas	Solid	Hydrogen in palladium
Liquid	Solid	Mineral oil in paraffin
Solid	Solid	Solder (tin in lead)

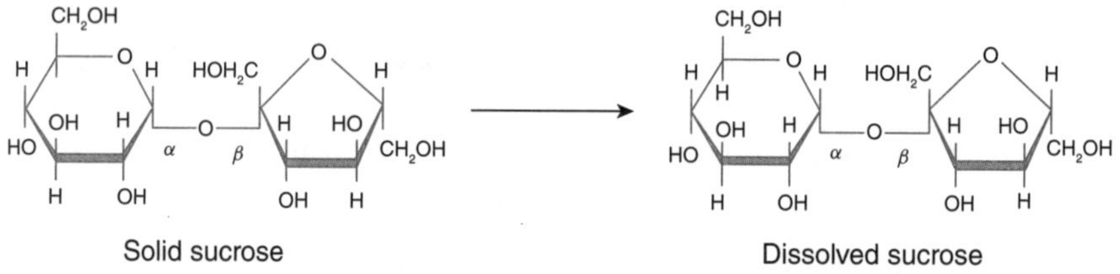

Solid sucrose → Dissolved sucrose

Figure 3.4 Dissolution when solute remains the same chemical entity

When sucrose dissolves in water it remains unchanged. When the solvent (water) is removed, sucrose is recovered.

In the situation described, dissolution occurs without the requirement of ionization. Thus, the intermolecular interactions discussed in Chapter 1 play prominent roles in the first type of dissolution.

For the second type of dissolution, the original solute is either not recoverable, or not completely recoverable. The resulting solution contains a compound that is different from that of the original solid phase. This change is generally due to some chemical reaction between the solute and solvent. When the solvent is removed, some or all of the solute is different from what was originally added to the solvent.

An example is that of (modern) 'aspirin' (acetylsalicylic acid) in plain water (Figure 3.5). While in solution, some of the aspirin hydrolyzes, forming acetic acid and salicylic acid. When water is removed, some of the original acetylsalicylic acid may be recovered, but also acetic and salicylic acids. Here, in order for dissolution to occur, the solute was required to ionize, and then the solvent was required to exert enough influence on the ions to overcome their cohesive forces.

Dissolution is a process

For either mode of dissolution, and in order for dissolution to occur – with or without an accompanying chemical reaction – the solute particle size is first

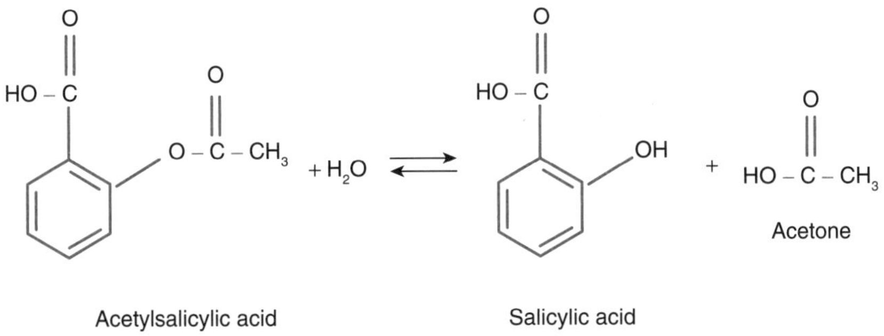

Figure 3.5 Dissolution when solute entity changes upon dissolution

When acetylsalicylic acid is dissolved in water some of it is hydrolyzed to salicylic acid and acetone. When the water is evaporated, not all of the recovered solute is in the original form of acetylsalicylic acid.

reduced. This initiates the process of dissolution. This process is measured as rate. The Noyes–Whitney equation describes dissolution in a single equation. But what occurs on a smaller scale? Solubility is now assumed, but we are now interested in how quickly the endpoint arrives. This can be a simple one-step consideration, with one associated rate, or dissolution can involve multiple steps, each with its own rate. The collection of individual rates results in an overall dissolution rate that we can observe.

As an introduction, a diagram of the dissolution of a tablet or capsule is illustrated below (Figure 3.6). For tablets and capsules there are three steps to dissolution. These three steps are disintegration, deaggregation, and dissolution. From any point (Figure 3.6), direct dissolution can occur, and in fact, all steps may be occurring simultaneously.

Key Point

Dissolution of a solid in a liquid often actually involves three steps:

- Disintegration
- Deaggregation
- Dissolution

Figure 3.7 illustrates the observations made for dissolution of a tablet if it followed the longest series of steps as outlined above.

If we were to look closely, even dissolution from a powder form can be a multi-step process. Depending on the solute particle size (degree of particle size reduction), the dissolution process of powders in solvent can be visualized as shown in Figure 3.8.

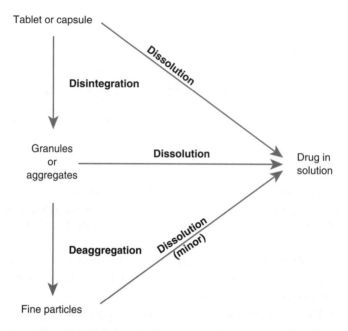

Figure 3.6 The dissolution process

The dissolution of a solid solute can be visualized as a general movement from the largest form, to granules or aggregates, then to fine particles, before becoming molecularly dispersed (dissolved). However, removal of molecules (dissolution) from the various steps of decreasing particle size can occur any time during the overall process.

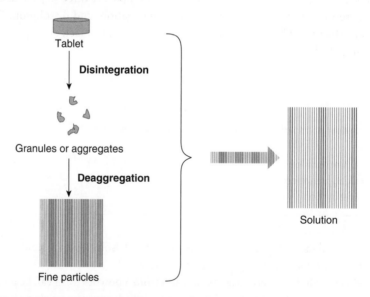

Figure 3.7 Disintegration, deaggregation, and the solution process

An illustration of the steps for tablet dissolution also shows how dissolution of various forms of solutes can occur. Though dissolution can occur from all forms of a solute (dosage form, granules/ aggregates or fine particles), the major path is through all three forms.

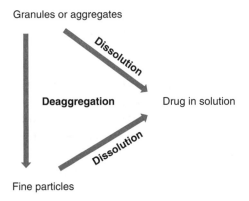

Figure 3.8 Process of dissolution restricted to smaller particles

If solute particles have been mechanically reduced (e.g., by trituration), the process of dissolution can be viewed as involving the lower portion of the scheme depicted in Figure 3.6.

Each of the steps of dissolution has its own rate. These rates can be expressed as dS/dt (solid to granules/aggregates), dG/dt (granules/aggregates to fine particles), dP/dt (particles to solution), and all the equations for individual steps to solution. Of course, each step can lead directly to dissolution, as previously stated. Visualizing this would lead to a rather complicated picture of these steps, as shown in Figure 3.9.

The sum of the equations would be quite unwieldy. Each step in Figure 3.9 is shown moving one direction, when each is truly an equilibrium equation. Most

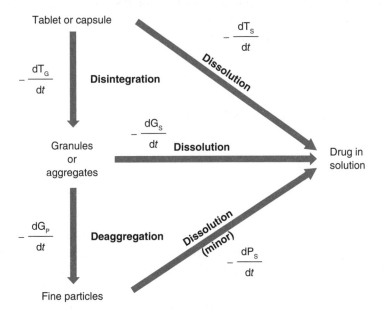

Figure 3.9 A mathematical scheme for dissolution

To consider all of the dissociation components, we would need to combine and summate $-dT_a/dt$, $-dG_p/dt$, $-dG_s/dt$, $-dT_s/dt$, and $-dP_s/dt$. This obviously would be very cumbersome.

of the processes occur as illustrated in Figure 3.8. The Noyes–Whitney equation helps us avoid complication by focusing on the most important step of dissolution: movement of fine particles into solution.

Therefore, this discussion will center on what occurs after the drug delivery system provides granules or aggregates ('chunks'). Of particular interest is what transpires with fine particles. Intermolecular interactions between the solvent and large 'chunks' of solute cause the solute to be reduced to fine particles. All the while, when solute particles have detached from the larger pieces, dissolution has been occurring. However, once the solute is reduced to fine particles, its increase in total available surface area lends to optimum interaction with the solvent. As the system/total particle size is reduced, the total solute surface area greatly increases. From the point that the solute has been reduced to fine particles, wetting – especially immersional wetting (discussed below) – is occurring. Wetting involves displacing air from the particle surface, along with creating effective interfacial contact between the solute and solvent.

Fine particles and wetting

If we now focus on only actions at the fine particle level, the process of fine particle dissolution can be thought of as following three steps. The first, as just mentioned, is wetting of the solute by the solvent. This is followed by immersion of the solute in the solvent, which involves not only favorable interfacial energetics, but also the thermodynamics discussed above. Finally, diffusion of molecules of solute into the bulk solution must occur (Figure 3.10).

Key Point

Fine particle dissolution follows these steps:

- Wetting
- Immersion
- Diffusion

Wetting: When preparing a solution using a solute powder and liquid solvent, slow wetting of the solute by the solvent can be a hindrance to what might otherwise be a quick and easy dissolution process. Physically, air pockets can be trapped inside the powder, slowing the initial ability of the powder to contact the solvent well. In addition, interfacial interactions are very important for dissolution – again intermolecular interactions are emphasized, this time with regard to solute, solvent and environmental interactions. The ability for a solvent to wet a solute is dependent on

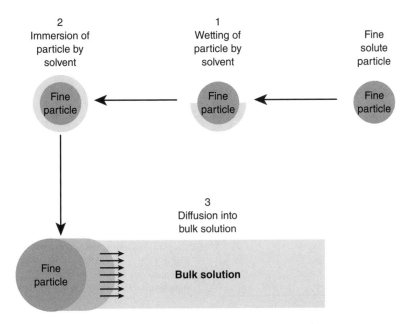

Figure 3.10   Three steps of fine solute dissolution

Once a solute is finely subdivided, there can conceptually be three steps toward dissolution: 1) wetting of the particles; 2) complete immersion of the particles; and 3) diffusion of particles into the bulk.

surface tension. Young's equation is a method of accounting for, and using, surface tension values to predict how easily a solute will be wetted, and ultimately dissolved. First, the solvent needs to spread over the surface of the solute. Then, the solvent needs to immerse the solute. Both of these steps, along with illustration of the parameters of Young's equation, are shown in Figure 3.11. Young's equation is:

$$\gamma_{S/A} = \gamma_{S/L} + \gamma_{L/A} \cos \theta$$

Since the value of θ will be between 0° and 90°, θ varies from 1 to 0, and $\gamma_{L/A}$ cos θ will be zero, or a positive value. $\gamma_{S/A}$ = surface tension of the solid at the solid–air boundary, $\gamma_{S/L}$ = solid–liquid interfacial tension, $\gamma_{L/A}$ = surface tension of the liquid–air boundary, and θ is the contact angle between the solid and liquid. If θ is less than zero, the substance is considered hydrophilic. If θ is greater than 90°, the substance is considered hydrophobic. When water is the solvent, a hydrophilic solute is desirable.

Key Point

Young's equation is used to calculate solute and solvent surface tension values, and explain and predict the wettability of the solute, and so is a predictor of ease of dissolution.

A

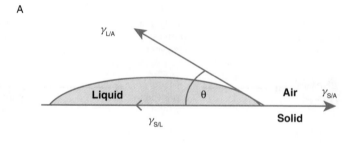

B

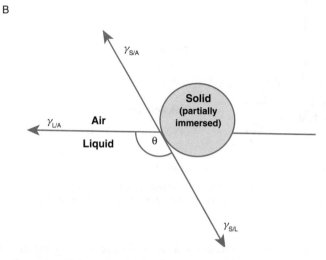

Figure 3.11 Illustration of the components of Young's equation

This figure illustrates the forces acting on (A) a liquid droplet on a solid surface and (B) the liquid on a partially immersed solid. (A) Initial spreading of the solvent over the solute: the components of Young's equation in relation to the particle surface (x-axis) and the wetting process are shown. (B) Spreading of the solvent over partially immersed solute: Young's equation extended to the immersion process is shown. $\gamma_{S/A}$, the surface tension between the solid and air; $\gamma_{L/A}$, between the liquid (solvent) and air; and $\gamma_{S/L}$, the inferred extension between solid and liquid (solvent).

For the initial step – spreading of the solvent over the solute – the spreading coefficient (S) is important:

$$S = \gamma_{L/A} (\cos \theta - 1)$$

Positive values for S indicate the solvent will completely spread over the surface of the solute, whereas negative values for S are indicative of difficulty in wetting the solute surface. If $(\cos \theta - 1)$ is positive, the value of S is positive and spreading of the solvent is favored. If $(\cos \theta - 1)$ is negative, the value of S is negative and the solvent spreading is unfavorable/unlikely. Spontaneous wetting occurs if the contact angle is $0°$ (Figure 3.12).

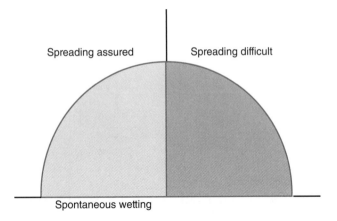

Figure 3.12 Prediction of liquid spreading on a particle surface based on particle–liquid contact angle, θ. If $\theta - 1$ = positive values, spontaneous spreading/wetting is predicted. For $\theta - 1$ = negative values, wetting is unfavorable.

Immersional wetting, the subsequent step to spreading (Figure 3.12), is also dictated by the angle the solute surface makes with the air–liquid interface.

Another way to approach the concept of wetting is shown in Figure 3.13. For solid–liquid systems, there are forces of adhesion and cohesion. As has been outlined above, the solid (solute) must be wetted by liquid before the solid can dissolve in it. In Figure 3.13(A), the solid is in contact with the liquid, so the energy existing between the solid and liquid can be defined using the interfacial free energy, or surface tension, $\gamma_{S/L}$, and adhesive work is proportional to the solid and liquid surface tensions, minus the solid–liquid interfacial tension. If the liquid and solid are conceptually separated, there are two surface tensions created: one between the solid and air ($\gamma_{S/A}$), the other between the liquid and the air ($\gamma_{L/A}$). The work of adhesion is proportional to the energy required to separate the liquid from the solid:

$$W_A = \gamma_{L/A} + \gamma_{S/A} - \gamma_{S/L}$$

In Figure 3.13(B), the liquid is in contact with the liquid (itself), so the energy existing between the liquid and liquid is the work of cohesion, because by separating the liquid from itself, two liquid–air interfaces are created, each with a surface tension ($\gamma_{L/A}$). There is no interfacial tension between the two liquid 'pieces' before separation because the liquid is a single phase. The work of cohesion then is:

$$W_C = \gamma_L + \gamma_L = 2\gamma_L$$

Simply put, if the work of adhesion exceeds the work of cohesion, wetting will tend to occur. Spreading of a liquid on a solid will occur when the work of

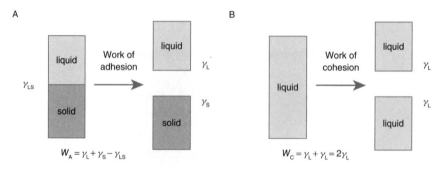

Figure 3.13 Concept of wetting

(A) illustrates the work of adhesion (W_A) between liquid (solvent) and solute; (B) illustrates the work of cohesion (W_c) within the solvent/liquid.

adhesion exceeds the work of cohesion. That is, spreading is favored when forces between different molecules exceed those between similar molecules.

$$W_A > W_C$$

S is the spreading coefficient. As stated above, when S is positive, the liquid will spread on the solid.

$$S = W_A - W_C$$

Substituting in for the variable, $S = \gamma_{L/L} + \gamma_{S/A} - \gamma_{S/L} - 2\gamma_{L/A}$.

$$S = \gamma_{S/A} - \gamma_{L/A} - \gamma_{S/L}.$$

Using either Young's equation or comparing adhesive and cohesive work, it can be seen that, in order to improve wetting, $\gamma_{S/A}$ and/or $\gamma_{S/L}$ must be reduced. This can be accomplished using surfactants. Surfactants, or 'surface active agents', reduce surface tension, allowing particle wetting more easily. Wetting of a solid can be an issue with any liquid dosage form, including solutions (Chapter 4), suspensions, and emulsions (Chapter 7), which will be discussed further. Thus, the wetting of the solute accomplished, the rest of the dissolution process continues – namely, diffusion.

Diffusion leads to solutions

Diffusion: To illustrate the diffusion process, the diffuse double layer (DDL) model was developed, which helps describe parameters responsible for the rate

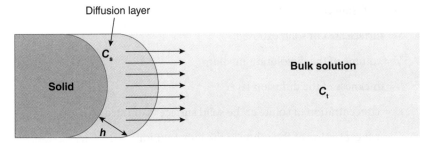

Figure 3.14   The diffuse double layer (DDL) model and diffusion

The DDL model can be utilized to account for characteristics of diffusion, the final step of the dissolution process.

of dissolution. The Noyes–Whitney equation below provides a mathematical description of the DDL model.

The DDL model is based on the Noyes–Whitney equation (Figure 3.1) and is illustrated in a slightly modified form in Figure 3.14. The model can be described as a solute surface immersed in solvent. When a solid dissolves, the components pass down a diffusion gradient (diffusion layer) until the particle completely dissolves and enters the bulk solution.

The variables in this model are as follows:

C_s = the concentration of solute in solvent very near the surface of the solute (solid). This is also the saturation concentration for the solute in the solvent;

C_t = the concentration of solute in the bulk solution;

h = the concentration gradient, or diffusion layer, through which the solute particles pass, on their way to the bulk solution.

The diffusion layer is thought of as a 'film' very near the solid surface. This film forms a thin stagnant layer (h) around the particle. At the particle surface the solution is saturated (C_s). Molecules first traverse through h almost instantaneously, then diffuse from h into the bulk solution. This diffusion step is slower and often rate limiting. The bulk solution has a concentration (C_t) that varies with time, until the dissolution process has been completed. The model illustrates rate of dissolution as an image. The Noyes–Whitney equation describes the model (Figure 3.14) mathematically:

$$\frac{dC}{dt} = \frac{Ds}{Vh}(C_s - C_t)$$

where

$$\frac{dC}{dt} = \text{Dissolution rate} = \frac{\dfrac{mg}{mL}}{\text{Change in time}}$$

D = diffusion coefficient of the solute in solution

S = surface area of solid exposed

V = volume of the dissolution medium

h = thickness of the diffusion layer

C_s = concentration of solute at the solid surface (saturated)

C_t = concentration of the solute in the bulk solution.

Key Point

The Noyes–Whitney equation describes dissolution, which includes diffusion. Diffusion is further described by the Stokes–Einstein equation.

Since diffusion is often rate limiting, it is of special importance within the Noyes–Whitney equation. In addition, the diffusion coefficient D is dependent on several parameters, including the Boltzmann constant, the absolute temperature, viscosity of the medium and radius of the solute molecule (which should be noted decreases as the solution process proceeds), and is described by the Stokes–Einstein equation:

$$D = \frac{kT}{6\pi\eta r}$$

where

D = diffusion coefficient of the solute in solution
k = Boltzmann constant
T = absolute temperature
η = viscosity of the solvent
r = radius of the solute molecule.

Inspection of the Noyes–Whitney and Stokes–Einstein equations reveals to us the parameters that can affect the dissolution rate of solutes in solvents. Some implications are intuitive. As the solution temperature increases, so does the diffusion coefficient, and so the dissolution rate increases. As the viscosity of the solvent increases, the dissolution rate decreases. As the radius of the solute decreases, total solute surface area increases, and dissolution rate increases. As the solute surface area increases, so does dissolution rate. So what might be some applications? If we can warm solvents, dissolution rate may be increased, depending on the nature of the solute. This 'if' is because care must be taken as for the potential for degradation of the solute at higher temperatures, so we must not blindly increase temperature without regard to the solute(s). Also, of course, there are some solutes whose solubility is not improved by increasing temperature. With regard to viscosity of the solvent or medium, we should be aware that solutes will tend to dissolve more slowly in more viscous solvents (e.g., syrups rather than water), and so it may be advisable to dissolve solutes in solvents prior to adding excipients that will increase the overall viscosity of the preparation. We cannot always alter the radius of the solute molecules (other than by trituration), but we can anticipate larger solute molecules will dissolve more slowly than smaller ones, and so expect more time for dissolution to go to completion. The thickness of the unstirred layer (h) can be decreased *in vitro*, such as by stirring in a beaker, thus increasing dissolution rate. The analogous action *in vivo* is less likely to be accomplished with much success. Perhaps if the patient were required to jump up and down after ingestion of the solute, one could show improved *in vivo* dissolution. Decreasing the solid surface area (S) increases dissolution rate, so subdivision/trituration of the solute prior to its addition to the solvent should improve dissolution rate. Regarding the saturation concentration of a solute: one must be careful not to indiscriminately elevate temperatures *in vitro*. Not only may this degrade the solute, as mentioned above, but also a supersaturated solution may be created. When this supersaturated solution is then cooled, the solute(s) may precipitate out of solution. With regard to the solute concentration at time $= t$ (C_t), it may be observed that, as the saturation concentration (C_s) is approached, dissolution will begin to slow down. The applications include making saturated solutions ahead of time because the last bit of dissolution may take a long time, and it may be advisable to maintain stock bottles of saturated solutions.

If it can be assumed the concentration beyond h is very small (perhaps, for calculations, equal to '0'), then the Noyes–Whitney equation simplifies to:

$$\frac{dC}{dt} = \frac{DS}{Vh}(C_s)$$

This may be the case when there is a large volume of bulk solvent or stirring effectively removes the DDL (h is nearly 0). When these occur, it is said sink conditions exist (i.e., the solute is disappearing as if 'going down a sink drain').

Summary

In summary, solubility and dissolution have been discussed. There are several important parameters that dictate a given solute's solubility in a given solvent. Once these parameters are understood and any optimizations made, the solubility of a solute must be understood to be an endpoint. On the other hand, dissolution is a study of the effects various parameters have on the rate at which a solute reaches its solubility.

Self-assessment questions

1. What is a solution?

2. Why do solubility and dissolution mean different things?

3. How can we influence solubility of a substance in a solvent?

4. How can we influence the process of dissolution?

5. Name the three main steps of tablet dissolution.

6. Fine particle dissolution follows what three-step process?

7. What contact angle (θ) is predictive of best – or most spontaneous – wetting?

8. What is a surfactant?

9. What is the DDL model?

10. In order for particle wetting to occur, what is true regarding work of adhesion and work of cohesion?

4

Colligative properties of solutions

Upon completion of this chapter, you should be able to answer the following questions:

- What is a colligative property?
- What are the four colligative properties?
- How are colligative properties related to preparation of drug delivery systems?
- What are the consequences of not taking into account colligative properties when calculating isotonicity?

Common liquid dosage forms

Solutions are the most common liquid drug delivery system, often employed for oral, parenteral, ophthalmic, otic, topical, vaginal, and rectal preparations. The term solution should not be confused with other liquid systems. A solution can be defined as a mixture of two or more substances, which is both chemically and physically homogeneous. Other, non-solution liquid dosage forms are heterogeneous and include disperse systems, which are discussed in Chapters 6 and 7. Once a solute completely dissolves in a solvent and a solution is formed, the solution acts as a single entity, with a single phase. Disperse systems contain two or more phases. Briefly, disperse systems are not solutions as the 'solute' is not truly dissolved, but rather is dispersed in the 'solvent.' In practice, the terms 'solute' and 'solvent' are (inaccurately) sometimes applied to 'dispersed phase' and 'dispersion medium' in a casual sense, but it is understood these are misnomers. In a disperse system, solid particles may be invisible to the eye, but are not truly in solution. Therefore, disperse systems have innate issues with regard to phase separation. Liquid systems are listed in order of increasing particle size in Table 4.1.

Other types of liquid delivery systems include colloids, suspensions, and emulsions, which will be discussed in Chapters 6 and 7. These liquid delivery systems are heterogeneous, and so always present the pharmacist with potential stability issues, mainly that of the components separating. Because solutions are

Table 4.1 Relative sizes of particles relevant to most drug delivery systems	
Liquid system	**In order of approximate increasing particle size (nm)**
Solutions	<1.0 nm
Disperse systems	
Colloidal dispersions ('colloids')	1.0–1000 nm
Coarse dispersions	100–50 000 nm
Suspensions	
Emulsions	

homogeneous, unless there are extraneous influences acting upon them, they are normally considered very stable once formed. The most important circumstances where solutions threaten to become unstable are: 1) when the solute concentration is near its saturation concentration; 2) when temperature fluctuations may cause solutes to precipitate out of solution; and 3) when pH changes occur.

Unless something disturbs a solution (e.g., extreme solute concentration or temperature), there is normally no reason to fear its stability, aside from potential microbial contamination. It should be remembered that the dissolution process is a dynamic equilibrium, meaning the dynamics of crystallization and solution must be complete, and the solute 'completely' in solution, in order for a solution to be useful. During the dissolution process, intermolecular interactions are once again at work. Solute particles attract each other; solvent particles also attract each other (cohesive interactions), but hopefully there is sufficient attraction between solute and solvent particles to favor some, or all, of the solute to dissolve. Arguably, the most important aspect regarding pharmaceutical application of solutions is the total solubility of the solute in the solvent. The next most important aspect is the dissolution rate of the solute in the solvent. For end products it is assumed dissolution is complete. However, when preparing solutions for drug use, the amount of time required for the solution to be 'ready' (thus, its dissolution rate) is tantamount, and often dissolution is the rate-limiting step when preparing solutions for drug delivery systems.

Colligative properties

Until this point, when 'solutions' have been discussed, it has been implied that, once a solute has dissolved into the solvent and a solution created, the solution then behaves in an ideal manner, meaning it could be assumed that physical attributes of the solution, like freezing point, remain the same for the solution. However, once again, intermolecular interactions cause deviations from anticipated behavior, and can affect the successful preparation or administration of various drug delivery systems.

Recall introductory chemistry: it may have been interesting to learn that the properties of freezing point, boiling point and vapor pressure of various substances could be altered by the addition of a second substance – an 'impurity.' Perhaps even the property of osmotic pressure, and the effects added solutes have on it, were discussed in this context. These are the four colligative properties of solutions. Colligative properties are those that depend on the number of particles in a solution, not the nature of the particles.

There are extensive and intensive physical properties for substances. Extensive properties include parameters such as mass and volume and depend on the amount, or size, of the substance being measured. Intensive properties include characteristics such as density and concentration, and are characteristics of the specific substance, regardless of how much of the substance is observed. Colligative properties are intensive properties of solutions. A formal definition for a colligative property is that the property depends on the quantity (or concentration) of particles in a solution, but is independent of the identity of the particles.

The colligative properties of a given solution include its vapor pressure, boiling point, freezing point and osmotic pressure. The phenomena associated with addition of solute to solvent are vapor pressure lowering, boiling point elevation, freezing point depression and osmotic pressure elevation (changes). All of these are induced by the added solute and result in deviations from properties of the pure solvent. The colligative property most identifiable with biological consequences is osmotic pressure. However, any colligative property can be used to observe (and also to calculate) the effects of addition of a solute to a solvent, and be equated to the other colligative properties. That is, they all indirectly tell us the same information regarding change in the solution, only they are telling us in different 'languages.' What are colligative properties, what causes them, and what are the applications with regard to pharmaceuticals?

Key Point

> Colligative property deviations that result from adding solute to pure solvent depend only on the amount of added solute, not what the substance added is.

How many particles?

Colligative properties of liquids are affected by the number of particles (molecules or ions) of the solute added to the liquid and are not dependent on the chemical character of the particles. The difficulty is to accurately account for the number of particles and this is not always as straightforward as it may appear. 'Particles' usually refers to molecules or ions. However, it is probably familiar that in many cases, solutes, especially electrolytes, though perhaps completely dissolved (by the definition provided in Chapter 3) are not always completely ionically dissociated. Ionization is an equilibrium process. This is important to us because colligative properties, being dependent on the number of particles in solutions, deviate from 'ideal' calculations when potentially ionizable solutes are included in a dosage form, but the deviations differ from what might be expected, even if we know precisely how much solute was added. This affects the quantities of solutes that are actually added to solutions. Thus, solutions we deal with will frequently deviate from ideal expectations and our cursory calculations. Whether deviations will exert enough impact on either the patient or the drug delivery system must be considered when preparing solutions – especially those for parenteral administration. Colligative properties, like many important aspects of drug delivery systems, result from intermolecular interactions, and we will briefly see why for each colligative property. With a little mathematical manipulation, all values can be related to concentration, and therefore number of particles, and so be practically applied to dosage form preparation. A brief overview of the four colligative properties is provided below.

The four colligative effects

Freezing point depression: By adding solute particles, the solvent is diluted, decreasing solvent–solvent interactions, and, ultimately, crystal formation. In order for the solution to freeze, a lower temperature must be attained than is required for freezing the pure solvent. Freezing point depression (ΔT_f) is calculated using the equation:

$$\Delta T_f = T_f \text{(solution)} - T_f \text{(solvent)} = K_f \times m$$

where T_f = freezing point, K_f is the cryoscopic constant (= 1.86°C kg/mol for water) and m = molality of the solution.

Boiling point elevation: As described above, dissolution of a solute, while increasing the concentration of the solute, can be viewed as diluting the concentration of solvent molecules, as well as establishing attractive forces between solvent and solute molecules. The result is a decreased tendency for solvent molecules to escape, or leave, the solution (i.e., evaporate or boil) compared with pure solvent. Therefore, a higher temperature must be attained by the solution than by the pure solvent in order to boil. Boiling point elevations (ΔT_b) are calculated by the equation:

$$\Delta T_b = T_b \text{(solution)} - T_b \text{(solvent)} = K_b \times m$$

where K_b is the ebullioscopic constant of the solvent (= 0.512°C kg/mol for water).

Vapor pressure depression: As occurs when other colligative properties are explained, dissolving a solute in a solvent decreases the solvent–solvent (cohesive) interactions, while increasing the solvent–solute (adhesive) interactions, resulting, as measured with vapor pressure, in a decreased tendency for solvent molecules to escape the solution, compared with the tendency for pure solvent. Vapor pressure is the force exerted above a liquid (or solid) that results from evaporation of a liquid (or solid) in a closed container. Fewer numbers of solvent molecules vaporizing, by definition, is decreased vapor pressure. Vapor pressure is governed by the parameters included in Raoult's law:

$$P_A = X_A P_A^0$$

where P_A = solution vapor pressure, P_A^0 = pure solvent vapor pressure, and X_A = mole fraction of solvent.

This shows that addition of a solute, B, to solvent A results in a decreased vapor pressure of solvent A. This form of Raoult's law focuses on the resulting mole fraction of the solvent but leaves us to further determine the amount of solute that is represented by subtracting from one. The colligative property of vapor pressure depression, resulting from the addition of a solute, B, is really what is of interest. That is, when a solute, X_B, is added to a solvent, how much is the vapor pressure decreased? This is simply looking directly at how the quantity of solute affects the solvent. If we know the mole fraction of the solute, X_B, then this can be calculated from:

$$\frac{P_A^0 - P_A}{P_A^0} = X_B$$

X_B will be a unitless fraction, which can then be converted to percent or to Pascals if desired. Therefore, if we are adding a known amount of solute, B, we can estimate what the magnitude of the resulting vapor pressure depression will be.

Osmotic pressure elevation: If a solute is dissolved in a solvent, the solvent's osmotic pressure is increased. Osmotic pressure is the force applied against a semipermeable membrane by a liquid. Adding solute to the liquid (solvent) can increase that force. If solutes are unable to cross the membrane, but solvents can, osmotic pressure on a membrane can be established, and measured. The lower the concentration of solvent, the higher the osmotic pressure. The higher the solute concentration, the more osmotic pressure is exerted, compared with that of pure solvent. The osmotic pressure of a solution is the difference in pressure between that exerted by the solution versus that of the pure solvent across a semipermeable membrane. In a way, osmotic pressure can be viewed as the resultant force (on the surrounding membrane) applied by a pure solvent, as it proceeds toward equilibrating solute concentration differences. Osmotic pressure change is calculated by the Morse equation:

$$\pi = RTm$$

where R = gas constant, T = absolute temperature, and m = molality of the solution.

Table 4.2 The four colligative property equations	
Colligative property	Equation
Vapor pressure lowering	$\Delta P = X_2 P_1$
Boiling point elevation	$\Delta T_b = K_b m$
Freezing point depression	$\Delta T_f = K_f m$
Osmotic pressure (elevation)	$\Pi = RTm$

Solutes that completely dissolve and do not ionize ('simple solutes') provide straightforward alterations in colligative properties. For these solutions, the four formulae above are accurate. But, what about solutes that have more than one species? These solutes require more attention because if they do not completely ionize, they act partly as the unionized species, but partly as whatever ionizable species may be available. Sometimes the number of species is complicated, and ultimately what is utilized is something of a 'weighted average' of each of the ionic forms that are present. But how do we know the proportion of each ionic species? This will be addressed below. A summary of the ideal colligative properties is provided in Table 4.2.

Electrolytes and deviations in colligative properties

Electrolytes are substances that dissolve in water, providing a solution that conducts electricity. An example is sodium chloride:

$$NaCl \rightleftharpoons Na^+ + Cl^-$$

To begin with, we will assume the ideal condition of 100% dissociation. It will be shown below why the assumption that a solution will behave ideally can lead to puzzling results, especially if the concepts are not understood. The term dissociation, as it is used pertaining to ions, should not be confused with dissociation of particles from a larger solid, as part of the dissolution process. Solutes capable of producing ions that have the capacity to conduct electricity meet the criteria for electrolytes. Electrolytes that are thought to completely (or nearly completely) dissociate are called strong electrolytes. Sodium chloride is a strong electrolyte. Electrolytes that are known to incompletely dissociate are called weak electrolytes. An example of a weak electrolyte is mercury chloride:

$$HgCl_2 \text{ (aq)} \xrightleftharpoons[]{2.55 \times 10^{-6} \text{ M}} HgCl^+ \text{ (aq)} + Cl^- \text{ (aq)}$$

Mercury chloride is highly polar but only a small amount (7.4% at 20°C) ionizes in water, meaning the solubility in water is 7.4 g/100 mL. A solution containing mercury chloride does conduct electricity, therefore it is an electrolyte. Keep in mind that dissolution and complete dissociation of ions are two different concepts. Silver chloride is poorly soluble but is a strong electrolyte. Water, as a solvent, does not dissolve a relatively large amount of silver chloride compared to that of sodium chloride. However, of the silver chloride that is dissolved, most of the Ag^+ and Cl^- completely dissociate from each other. Solutes that dissolve in water but are not fragmented into ions (i.e., maintain their molecular structure in solution), do not conduct electricity and are called nonelectrolytes. An example of a nonelectrolyte is glucose. The dissolution of glucose ($C_6H_{12}O_6$) in water:

$$C_6H_{12}O_6 \rightleftharpoons C_6H_{12}O_6 \text{ (dissolution, but no dissociation)}$$

Key Point

Electrolytes cannot be assumed to dissociate, even if they dissolve. The actual extent of an electrolyte dissociation results in a different number of particles present from the number expected if complete dissociation is assumed.

As a general rule, it may be assumed that most strong electrolytes in solution are actually only about 80% dissociated. The remaining 20% is present in associated forms, such as ion pairs (Figure 4.1). The use of 80% dissociation is a generalization that works for most practical applications. It is emphasized that this is not exact. This 'rule' is based on the work of van't Hoff and others, which is generalized to commonly used electrolytes in pharmaceuticals.

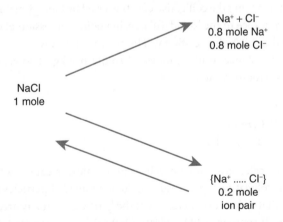

Figure 4.1 Explanation of van't Hoff i values correction for electrolyte dissociation

van't Hoff (and others) noted deviations from ideal dissociation could be explained using the concept of ion pairs as a reservoir for a portion of what previously was believed to be dissociated electrolyte. The application was to determine corrected dissociation constants for various electrolytes. These values often are labeled E in tables.

One mole of sodium chloride results in 1.8 moles of particles (Figure 4.1), rather than the predicted two moles. This deviation from expectation will impact the accuracy of calculations pertaining to drug solutions, as will be illustrated below. First, the application of colligative properties to solutions will be reviewed.

Colligative properties applied to pharmaceutical solutions

An example, using freezing point depression is: 'How much sodium chloride would be required to be added to 100 mL of water to depress the freezing point 0.52°C if the sodium chloride is completely dissociated?' To begin, the 'complete dissociation' of sodium chloride assumption allows for a simple calculation as complete dissociation of sodium chloride provides two particles from the initial one. The value selected for the freezing point depression chosen is significant because this is actually the freezing point of blood. That is, blood exhibits a freezing point depression of 0.52°C compared to water. Why is the freezing point of blood of interest? Because matching colligative actions of pharmaceutical liquids causes them to act in a 'physiologic' way with regard to tonicity. Tonicity is the amount of pressure exerted by a fluid against biological membranes. Ultimately, solutions we make for drug delivery systems usually need to be isotonic. Isotonic solutions are those that exert the same (osmotic) pressure against membranes as physiologic liquids do. Usually, the liquid we attempt to 'match' is the tonicity of blood. As mentioned previously, though it may initially seem odd to be associating freezing point with tonicity/osmotic pressure, all four colligative properties are interchangeable, and thus the inference of equivalence among them with regard to tonicity effects on solutions; therefore, the significance of matching the colligative effects exerted by biological fluids (e.g., cells) and so the significance of the 'standard' freezing point depression of 0.52°C. This is straightforward as 100% dissociation will be assumed for now:

m is the molal concentration, moles of solute per kg of solvent; 1.86° is the cryoscopic constant for water.

$$\Delta T_f = K_f m$$
$$0.52 = (1.86°C/m)m$$
$$m = 0.280 \text{ moles particles/L}$$

The result of calculating how much sodium chloride causes water to behave like blood in a colligative sense, results in '0.280 moles of particles per liter.' The implication is that it does not matter what the 'particles' actually are, just that they are in solution. If so, then 0.280 moles/L (280 mM) is a 'standard' for any solute in water, if we want the solution to behave like blood, with regard to osmotic pressure. Therefore, 0.280 moles of any particles/L provides 'physiologic osmotic pressure.' This is the concentration of particles in physiological fluids, and so the ideal for parenteral medication solutions.

Key Point

0.280 moles/L (280 mmol/L) of any solute, or combination of solutes, is considered isotonic.

The general method for matching 0.280 moles of particles per liter is to utilize the following ratio:

$$\frac{\text{MW of 1 mole of particles}}{1.86°C} = \frac{x}{0.52°C}$$

where x = weight (g) of solute needed to 'match' the freezing point depression, and so tonicity, of blood.

As an example, using sodium chloride:

$$1 \text{ mol NaCl} = \frac{58.443\text{g NaCl}/\text{mol NaCl}}{1.86°C} = \frac{x\text{g NaCl}/\text{L}}{0.52°C}$$

$$x = 16.338\text{g } (Na^+ + Cl^-, \text{ two particles}) = 8.169 \text{ g of NaCl}$$

Since we are assuming sodium chloride simply dissociates into Na^+ and Cl^-, giving 2 moles of particles, we need to adjust to a per mole basis by dividing by 2:

$$x = 16.338; \ x/2 = 8.169 \text{ g NaCl}$$

$$\frac{16.338\text{g NaCl}}{58.443 \text{ g}/\text{mol}} = 0.280 \text{ moles NaCl}$$

Since $NaCl = Na^+ + Cl^-$, this represents 0.280 moles of Na^+ and 0.280 moles Cl^-. Therefore, it was necessary to divide by 2.

van't Hoff's correction

Fortunately, rather than completing this arduous calculation for every solution prepared, we can use dissociation correction factors for various substances that have been determined by van't Hoff and others. In this text, the correction factor is represented as i, but in many reference tables it is referred to as E. The correction factors help account for incomplete dissociation, and so result in more accurate tonicity predictions. A portion of such a table is illustrated in Table 4.3.

Table 4.3 Examples of van't Hoff *i* correction values

		0.5 %		1 %		2 %		3 %		5 %		Iso-Osmotic Concentration[a]			
	E	D	E	D	E	D	E	D	E	D	%	E	D	H	pH
Acetrizoate methylglucamine	0.09		0.08		0.08		0.08		0.08	12.12	0.07			0	7.1
Acetrizoate sodium	0.10	0.027	0.10	0.055	0.10	0.109	0.10	0.163	0.10	0.273	9.64	0.09	0.52	0	6.9†
Acetrizoate sodium	0.10	0.027	0.10	0.055	0.10	0.109	0.10	0.163	0.10	0.273	9.64	0.09	0.52	0	6.9†
Adrenaline HCl											4.24			68	4.5
Alphaprodine HCl	0.19	0.053	0.19	0.105	0.18	0.212	0.18	0.315			4.98	0.18	0.52	100	5.3
Alum (potassium)			0.18				0.15		0.15		6.35		0.14	24*	3.4
Amantadine HCl	0.31	0.090	0.310	0.180	0.31	0.354					2.95	0.31	0.52	91	5.7
Aminoacetic acid	0.42	0.119	0.41	0.235	0.41	0.47					2.20	0.41	0.52	0*	6.2
Aminohippuric acid	0.13	0.035	0.13	0.075											
Aminophylline				0.098[c]											
Ammonium carbonate	0.70	0.202	0.70	0.405							1.29	0.70	0.52	97	7.7
Ammonium chloride			1.12								0.8	1.12	0.52	93	5.0
Ammonium lactate	0.33	0.093	0.33	0.185	0.33	0.37					2.76	0.33	0.52	98	5.9
Ammonium nitrate	0.69	0.200	0.69	0.400							1.30	0.69	0.52	91	5.3
Ammonium phosphate, dibasic	0.58	0.165	0.55	0.315							1.76	0.51	0.52	0	7.9
Ammonium sulfate	0.55	0.158	0.55	0.315							1.68	0.54	0.52	0	5.3
Amobarbital sodium			0.25	0.143[c]			0.25				3.6	0.25	0.52	0	9.3
D-Amphetamine HCl											2.64			98	5.7
Amphetamine phosphate			0.34	0.20			0.27	0.47			3.47	0.26	0.52	0	4.5
Amphetamine sulfate			0.22	0.129[c]			0.21	0.36			4.23	0.21	0.52	0	5.9
Amprotropine phosphate											5.90			0	4.2
Amylcaine HCl			0.22				0.19				4.98	0.18		100	5.6

Anileridine HCl	0.19	0.052	0.19	0.104	0.19	0.212	0.18	0.316	0.18	0.509	5.13	0.18	0.52	12	2.6
Antazoline phosphate							0.13				6.05			90	4.0
Antimony potassium tartrate			0.18						0.10			0.13			
Antipyrine			0.17	0.10	0.17		0.14	0.24	0.14	0.40	6.81		0.52	100	6.1
Apomorphine HCl	0.17		0.14	0.080c											
Arginine glutamate	0.17	0.048	0.17	0.097	0.17	0.195	0.17	0.292	0.17	0.487	5.37	0.17	0.52	0	6.9
Ascorbic acid				0.105c							5.05	0.52b	100*	2.2	
Atropine methylbromide			0.14				0.13		0.13		7.03	0.13			
Atropine methylnitrate											6.52			0	5.2
Atropine sulfate			0.13	0.075			0.11	0.19	0.11	0.32	8.85	0.10	0.52	0	5.0
Bacitracin			0.05	0.03			0.04	0.07	0.04	0.12					
Barbital sodium			0.30	0.171c			0.29	0.50			3.12	0.29	0.52	0	9.8
Benzalkonium chloride			0.16				0.14		0.13						
Benztropine mesylate	0.26	0.073	0.21	0.115	0.15	0.170	0.12	0.203	0.09	0.242					
Benzyl alcohol			0.17	0.09c			0.15								
Bethanechol chloride	0.50	0.140	0.39	0.225	0.32	0.368	0.30	0.512			3.05	0.30		0	6.0
Bismuth potassium tartrate			0.09				0.06		0.05						
Bismuth sodium tartrate			0.13				0.12		0.11		8.91	0.10		0	6.1
Boric acid	0.50	0.288c									1.9	0.47	0.52	100	4.6
Brompheniramine maleate	0.10	0.026	0.09	0.05	0.08	0.084									
Bupivacaine HCl	0.17	0.048	0.17	0.096	0.17	0.193	0.17	0.29	0.17	0.484	5.38	0.17	0.52	83	6.8
Butabarbital sodium	0.27	0.078	0.27	0.155	0.27	0.313	0.27	0.47			3.33	0.27	0.52	0	6.8

(continued)

Table 4.3 *(continued)*

	0.5 %		1 %		2 %		3 %		5 %		Iso-Osmotic Concentration[a]				
	E	D	E	D	E	D	E	D	E	D	%	E	D	H	pH
Butacaine sulfate			0.20	0.12	0.13		0.10	0.23		0.29	3.92	0.23	0.52	0	7.0
Caffeine and sodium benzoate			0.26	0.15	0.23			0.40			5.77	0.16	0.52	0	6.8
Caffeine and sodium salicylate			0.12	0.12	0.17		0.16	0.295	0.16	0.46				0	6.0
Calcium aminosalicylate											4.80				
Calcium chloride			0.51	0.298[c]							1.70	0.53	0.52	0	5.6
Calcium chloride (6H$_2$O)			0.35	0.20							2.5	0.36	0.52	0	5.7
Calcium chloride, anhydrous			0.68	0.39							1.3	0.69	0.52	0	5.6
Calcium disodium edetate	0.21	0.061	0.21	0.120	0.20	0.240		0.357			4.50	0.20	0.52	0	6.1
Calcium gluconate			0.16	0.091[c]	0.14			0.24							
Calcium lactate			0.23	0.13	0.12			0.36			4.5	0.20	0.52	0	6.7
Calcium lactobionate	0.08	0.022	0.08	0.043	0.07	0.085	0.07	0.126		0.197					
Calcium levulinate			0.27	0.16	0.25			0.43			3.58			0	7.2
Calcium pantothenate			0.129								5.50			0	7.4
Camphor			0.12[d]												
Capreomycin sulfate	0.04	0.011	0.04	0.02	0.04	0.042	0.04	0.063		0.106					
Carbachol			0.20	0.205[c]							2.82			0	5.9
Carbenicillin sodium	0.20	0.059	0.20	0.118	0.20	0.236		0.355			4.40	0.20	0.52	0	6.6
Carboxymethylcellulose sodium	0.03	0.007	0.145	0.017											
Cephaloridine	0.09	0.023	0.07	0.041	0.06	0.074	0.05	0.106							

Chloramine-T	0.14										4.10	0.13	0.52	100*	9.1
Chloramphenicol				0.06[d]											
Chloramphenicol sodium succinate	0.24	0.038	0.14	0.078	0.14	0.154	0.13	0.230	0.13	0.382	6.83	0.16	0.52	partial	6.1
Chlordiazepoxide HCl		0.068	0.22	0.125	0.19	0.220	0.18	0.315	0.17	0.487	5.50	0.16	0.52	66	2.7
Chlorobutanol (hydrated)	0.20		0.24	0.14	0.18	0.21									
Chloroprocaine HCl	0.14	0.054	0.20	0.108											
Chloroquine phosphate	0.10	0.039	0.14	0.082	0.14	0.162	0.14	0.242	0.13	0.379	7.15	0.13	0.52	0	4.3
Chloroquine sulfate		0.028	0.09	0.050	0.08	0.090	0.07	0.127	0.07	0.195					
Chlorpheniramine maleate	0.17	0.048	0.15	0.085	0.14	0.165	0.13	0.22	0.09	0.265					
Chlortetracycline HCl	0.10	0.030	0.10	0.061	0.10	0.121	0.10								
Chlortetracycline sulfate			0.13	0.08			0.17	0.17							
Citric acid			0.18	0.10				0.295	0.16	0.46	5.52	0.16	0.52	100*	1.8
Clindamycin phosphate	0.08	0.022	0.08	0.046	0.08	0.095	0.08	0.144	0.08	0.242	10.73	0.08	0.52	58*	6.8
Cocaine HCl			0.16	0.090[c]			0.15	0.26	0.14	0.40	6.33	0.14	0.52	47	4.4
Codeine phosphate			0.14	0.080[c]			0.13	0.23	0.13	0.38	7.29	0.12	0.52	0	4.4
Colistimethate sodium	0.15	0.045	0.15	0.085	0.15	0.170	0.15	0.253	0.14	0.411	6.73	0.13	0.52	0	7.6
Cupric sulfate			0.18	0.100[c]			0.15		0.14		6.85	0.13		trace*	3.9
Cyclizine HCl	0.20	0.060			0.10	0.125									
Cyclophosphamide	0.10	0.031	0.10	0.061	0.11	0.134	0.11	0.198	0.11	0.317	8.92	0.10	0.52	0	8.0
Cytarabine	0.11	0.034	0.11	0.066											
Deferoxamine mesylate	0.09	0.023	0.09	0.047	0.09	-0.093	0.09	0.142	0.09	0.241					
Demecarium bromide	0.14	0.038	0.12	0.069	0.10	0.108	0.08	0.139	0.07	0.192					

(continued)

Table 4.3 (continued)

	0.5%		1%		2%		3%		5%		Iso-Osmotic Concentration[a]				
	E	D	E	D	E	D	E	D	E	D	%	E	D	H	pH
Dexamethasone sodium phosphate	0.18	0.050	0.17	0.095	0.16	0.18	0.15	0.260	0.14	0.410	6.75	0.13	0.52	0	8.9
Dextroamphetamine HCl	0.34	0.097	0.34	0.196	0.34	0.392					2.64	0.34	0.52		
Dextroamphetamine phosphate	0.25		0.25	0.14	0.25			0.44			3.62	0.25	0.52	0	4.7
Dextroamphetamine sulfate	0.24	0.069	0.22	0.134	0.22	0.259	0.22	0.380			4.16	0.22	0.52	0	5.9
Dextrose				0.091[c]			0.16	0.28	0.16	0.46	5.51	0.16	0.52	0	5.9
Dextrose (anhydrous)				0.101[c]			0.18	0.31			5.05	0.18	0.52	0	6.0
Diatrizoate sodium	0.10	0.025	0.09	0.049	0.09	0.098	0.09	0.149	0.09	0.248	10.55	0.09	0.52	0	7.9
Dibucaine HCl				0.074[c]											
Dicloxacillin sodium (1H_2O)	0.10	0.030	0.10	0.061	0.10	0.122	0.10	0.182							
Diethanolamine	0.31	0.089	0.31	0.177	0.31	0.358					2.90	0.31	0.52	100	11.3
Dihydrostreptomycin sulfate	0.06		0.06	0.03	0.05		0.05	0.09	0.05	0.14	19.4	0.05	0.52	0	6.1
Dimethylpyrindene maleate	0.13	0.039	0.11	0.07	0.11	0.12									
Dimethyl sulfoxide	0.42	0.122	0.42	0.245	0.42	0.480					2.16	0.42	0.52	100	7.6
Diperodon HCl	0.15	0.045	0.14	0.079	0.13	0.141									
Diphenhydramine HCl	0.16	0.045	0.22	0.161[c]							5.70			88*	5.5
Diphenidol HCl	0.16	0.035	0.12	0.070	0.16	0.180									
Doxapram HCl	0.12	0.035	0.12	0.070	0.12	0.140	0.12	0.210							
Doxycycline hyclate	0.12	0.035	0.12	0.072	0.12	0.134	0.11	0.186	0.09	0.264					
Dyphylline	0.10	0.025	0.09	0.052	0.09	0.104	0.09	0.155	0.08	0.245					
Echothiophate iodide	0.16	0.045	0.16	0.090	0.16	0.179									
Edetate disodium	0.24	0.070	0.23	0.132	0.21	0.248	0.21	0.360			4.44	0.20	0.52	0	4.7
Edetate trisodium monohydrate	0.29	0.079	0.29	0.158	0.27	0.316	0.27	0.472			3.31	0.27	0.52	0	8.0

Emetine HCl	0.08			0.058[c]		0.28	0.17		0.29	3.2	0.28		96	5.9
Ephedrine HCl			0.30	0.165[c]		0.20	0.35			4.54	0.20	0.52	0	5.7
Ephedrine sulfate			0.23	0.13		0.16	0.28			5.7	0.16	0.52	100*	3.4
Epinephrine bitartrate			0.18	0.104		0.16	0.28		0.462					
Epinephrine hydrochloride			0.29	0.16[b]		0.26				3.47	0.26			
Ergonovine maleate				0.089[c]										
Erythromycin lactobionate		0.020	0.07	0.040	0.078	0.07	0.115	0.06	0.187					
Ethyl alcohol										1.39			100	6.0
Ethylenediamine				0.253[c]						2.08			100*	11.4
Ethylmorphine HCl			0.16	0.088[c]		0.15	0.26		0.43	6.18	0.15	0.52	38	4.7
Eucatropine HCl				0.11[d]										
Ferric ammonium citrate (green)										6.83			0	5.2
Floxuridine	0.14	0.040	0.13	0.076	0.147	0.12	0.213		0.335	8.47	0.12	0.52	3*	4.5
Fluorescein sodium		0.041	0.31	0.181[c]		0.27	0.47			3.34	0.27	0.52	0	8.7
Fluphenazine 2HCl	0.14		0.14	0.082	0.145	0.09	0.155							
D-Fructose										5.05			0*	5.9
Furtrethonium iodide	0.24	0.070	0.24	0.133	0.250	0.21	0.360			4.44	0.20	0.52	0	5.4
Galactose										4.92			0	5.9
Gentamicin sulfate	0.05	0.015	0.05	0.030	0.060	0.05	0.093		0.153					
D-Glucuronic acid										5.02			48*	1.6
Glycerin			0.203[c]						2.6			100	5.9	
Glycopyrrolate	0.15	0.042	0.15	0.084	0.166	0.14	0.242	0.13	0.381	7.22	0.12	0.52	92*	4.0
Gold sodium thiomalate	0.10	0.032	0.10	0.061	0.111	0.09	0.159	0.09	0.250					
Hetacillin potassium	0.17	0.048	0.17	0.095	0.190	0.17	0.284	0.17	0.474	5.50	0.17	0.52	0	
Hexafluorenium bromide	0.12	0.033	0.11	0.065									0	6.3

(continued)

Table 4.3 *(continued)*

Substance	E	0.5%		1%		2%		3%		5%		Iso-Osmotic Concentration[a]				
		D	E	D	E	D	E	D	E	D	E	%	E	D	H	pH
Hexamethonium tartrate	0.16	0.045	0.16	0.089	0.16	0.181	0.16	0.271	0.16	0.456	0.16	5.68	0.16	0.52		
Hexamethylene sodium acetaminosalicylate	0.18	0.049	0.18	0.099	0.17	0.199	0.17	0.297	0.16	0.485	0.16	5.48	0.16	0.52	0*	4.0
Hexobarbital sodium				0.15[c]												
Hexylcaine HCl												4.30			100	4.8
Histamine 2HCl	0.40	0.115	0.40	0.233	0.40	0.466						2.24	0.40	0.52	79*	3.7
Histamine phosphate				0.149[c]								4.10	0	4.6		
Histidine HCl												3.45			40	3.9
Holocaine HCl	0.20		0.20	0.12												
Homatropine hydrobromide	0.17		0.17	0.097[c]	0.16		0.16	0.28	0.16	0.46	0.16	5.67	0.16	0.52	92	5.0
Homatropine methylbromide	0.19		0.19	0.11			0.15	0.26		0.38	0.13					
4-Homosulfanilamide HCl												3.69			0	4.9
Hyaluronidase	0.01	0.004	0.01	0.007	0.01	0.013	0.01	0.02	0.01	0.033	0.01					
Hydromorphone HCl												6.39			64	5.6
Hydroxyamphetamine HBr				0.15[d]								3.71			92	5.0
8-Hydroxyquinoline sulfate												9.75			59*	2.5
Hydroxystilbamidine isethionate	0.20	0.06	0.16	0.090	0.12	0.137	0.10	0.17	0.07	0.216						
Hyoscyamine hydrobromide												6.53			68	5.9
Imipramine HCl	0.20	0.058	0.20	0.110		0.143	0.13									
Indigotindisulfonate sodium	0.30	0.085	0.30	0.172												

Intracaine HCl	0.18							4.97				85	5.0
Iodophthalein sodium			0.07c					9.58				100	9.4
Isometheptene mucate	0.14	0.048	0.095	0.18	0.196	0.18	0.302	4.95		0.18	0.52	0	6.2
Isoproterenol sulfate	0.14	0.039	0.078	0.14	0.156	0.14	0.234	6.65	0.389	0.14	0.52	trace	4.5
Kanamycin sulfate	0.08	0.021	0.041	0.07	0.083	0.07	0.125		0.210	0.07			
Lactic acid			0.239c					2.30				100*	2.1
Lactose	0.07		0.040c	0.08		0.08		9.75		0.09		0*	5.8
Levallorphan tartrate	0.13	0.036	0.073	0.13	0.143	0.12	0.210	9.40	0.329	0.10	0.52	59*	6.9
Levorphanol tartrate	0.12	0.033	0.067	0.12	0.136	0.12	0.203						
Lidocaine HCl	0.16		0.13c	0.15	0.170	0.14	0.247	4.42		0.14	0.52	85	4.3
Lincomycin HCl		0.045	0.090			0.14		6.60	0.40	0.14	0.52	0	4.5
Lobeline HCl			0.090*										
Lyapolate sodium	0.10	0.025	0.051	0.09	0.103	0.09	0.157	9.96	0.263	0.09	0.52	0	6.5+
Magnesium chloride			0.45					2.02		0.45		0	6.3
Magnesium sulfate	0.17		0.094c	0.15		0.15	0.26	6.3	0.43	0.14	0.52	0	6.2
Magnesium sulfate, anhydrous	0.34	0.093	0.184	0.30	0.345	0.29	0.495	3.18		0.28	0.52	0	7.0
Mannitol			0.098c						5.07		0*	6.2	
Maphenide HCl	0.075	0.27	0.27	0.153	0.27	0.303	0.26	3.55	0.448	0.25	0.52		
Menadiol sodium diphosphate								4.36				0	8.2
Menadione sodium bisulfite			0.12d					5.07				0	5.3
Menthol			0.125c										
Meperidine HCl									4.80			98	5.0
Mepivacaine HCl	0.21	0.060	0.116	0.20	0.230	0.20	0.342	4.60		0.20	0.52	45	4.5

(continued)

Table 4.3   (continued)

	0.5 %		1 %		2 %		3 %		5 %		%	Iso-Osmotic Concentration[a]			
	E	D	E	D	E	D	E	D	E	D		E	D	H	pH
Merbromin	0.10			0.08[b]											
Mercuric cyanide	0.15			0.06*	0.14		0.13								
Mersalyl															
Mesoridazine besylate	0.07	0.024	0.05	0.04	0.04	0.058	0.04	0.071		0.087					
Metaraminol bitartrate	0.20	0.06	0.20	0.112	0.18	0.21	0.17	0.308		0.505	5.17	0.17	0.52	59	3.8
Methacholine chloride				0.184[c]							3.21			0	4.5
Methadone HCl				0.101[c]							8.59			100*	5.0
Methamphetamine HCl				0.213[c]							2.75			97	5.9
Methdilazine HCl	0.12	0.035	0.10	0.056	0.08	0.08	0.06	0.093	0.04	0.112					
Methenamine	0.23		0.24		0.24		0.24				3.68	0.25		100	8.4
Methiodal sodium	0.24	0.068	0.24	0.136	0.24	0.274	0.24	0.41			3.81	0.24	0.52	0	5.9
Methitural sodium	0.26	0.074	0.25	0.142	0.23	0.275	0.23	0.407	0.16	0.453	3.85	0.23	0.52	78	9.8
Methocarbamol	0.10	0.03	0.10	0.06											
Methotrimeprazine HCl	0.12	0.034	0.10	0.060	0.07	0.077	0.06	0.094	0.04	0.125					
Methoxyphenamine HCl	0.26	0.075	0.26	0.150	0.26	0.300	0.26	0.450			3.47	0.26	0.52	96	5.4
p-Methylaminoethanol-phenol tartrate	0.18	0.048	0.17	0.095	0.16	0.19	0.16	0.282			5.83	0.16	0.52	0	6.2
Methyldopate HCl	0.21	0.063	0.21	0.122	0.21	0.244	0.21	0.365			4.28	0.21	0.52	partial	3.0
Methylergonovine maleate	0.10	0.028	0.10	0.056											
N-Methylglucamine	0.20	0.057	0.20	0.111	0.18	0.214	0.18	0.315			5.02	0.18	0.52	4	11.3
Methylphenidate HCl	0.22	0.065	0.22	0.127	0.22	0.258	0.22	0.388			4.07	0.22	0.52	66	4.3

Methylprednisolone Na succinate	0.10	0.025	0.09	0.051	0.09	0.102	0.08	0.143	0.07	0.20					
Minocycline HCl	0.10	0.030	0.10	0.058	0.09	0.107	0.08	0.146							
Monoethanolamine	0.53	0.154	0.53	0.306							1.70	0.53	0.52	100	11.4
Morphine HCl			0.15	0.086[c]			0.14								
Morphine sulfate			0.14	0.079[c]			0.11	0.19	0.09	0.26					
Nalorphine HCl	0.24	0.07	0.21	0.121	0.18	0.210	0.17	0.288	0.15	0.434	6.36	0.14	0.52	63	4.1
Naloxone HCl	0.14	0.042	0.14	0.083	0.14	0.158	0.13	0.230	0.13	0.367	8.07	0.11	0.52	35	5.2
Naphazoline HCl			0.27	0.14[d]			0.24				3.99	0.22		100	5.3
Neoarsphenamine											2.32		17	7.80	
Neomycin sulfate			0.11	0.063[c]			0.09	0.16	0.08	0.232					
Neostigmine bromide			0.22	0.127[c]			0.19				4.98			0	4.6
Neostigmine methylsulfate			0.20	0.115[c]			0.18		0.17		5.22	0.17			
Nicotinamide			0.26	0.148[c]			0.21	0.36			4.49	0.20	0.52	100	7.0
Nicotinic acid			0.25	0.144[c]											
Nikethamide				0.100[c]							5.94			100	6.9
Novobiocin sodium	0.12	0.033	0.10	0.057	0.07	0.073									
Oleandomycin phosphate	0.08	0.017	0.08	0.038	0.08	0.084	0.08	0.129	0.08	0.255	10.82	0.08	0.52	0	5.0
Orphenadrine citrate	0.13	0.037	0.13	0.074	0.13	0.144	0.12	0.204	0.10	0.285					
Oxophenarsine HCl											.67			trace*	2.3
Oxymetazoline HCl	0.22	0.063	0.22	0.124	0.20	0.232	0.19	0.335			4.92	0.18	0.52	86	5.7
Oxyquinoline sulfate	0.24	0.068	0.21	0.113	0.16	0.182	0.14	0.236	0.11	0.315		0.16			
D-Pantothenyl alcohol	0.20	0.053	0.18	0.100	0.17	0.193	0.17	0.283	0.16	0.468	5.60	0.16	0.52	92	6.8
Papaverine HCl			0.10	0.061[c]											

(continued)

Table 4.3 (continued)

	0.5 %		1 %		2 %		3 %		5 %		Iso-Osmotic Concentration[a]				
	E	D	E	D	E	D	E	D	E	D	%	E	D	H	pH
Paraldehyde	0.25	0.071	0.25	0.142	0.25	0.288	0.25	0.430			3.65	0.25	0.52	97	5.3
Pargyline HCl	0.30	0.083	0.29	0.165	0.28	0.327	0.28	0.491			3.18	0.28	0.52	91	3.8
Penicillin G, potassium			0.18	0.102[c]			0.16	0.29	0.16	0.46	5.48	0.16	0.52	0	6.2
Penicillin G, procaine				0.06[d]											
Penicillin G, sodium	0.15	0.042	0.18	0.100[c]		0.169	0.16	0.28	0.16	0.46	5.90			18	5.2
Pentazocine lactate			0.15	0.085			0.15	0.253	0.15	0.42					
Pentobarbital sodium				0.145[c]							4.07			0	9.9
Pentolinium tartrate				0.09[d]							5.95			55*	3.4
Phenacaine HCl				0.09											
Pheniramine maleate				0.09[d]											
Phenobarbital sodium			0.24	0.135[c]			0.23	0.40			3.95	0.23	0.52	0	9.2
Phenol	0.35	0.20									2.8	0.32	0.52	0*	5.6
Phentolamine mesylate	0.18	0.052	0.17	0.096		0.173	0.14	0.244	0.13	0.364	8.23	0.11	0.52	83	3.5
Phenylephrine HCl			0.32	0.184[c]							3.0	0.30		0	4.5
Phenylephrine tartrate											5.90			58*	5.4
Phenylethyl alcohol	0.25	0.070	0.25	0.141	0.25	0.283									
Phenylpropanolamine HCl			0.38	0.219[c]							2.6	0.35		95	5.3
Physostigmine salicylate			0.16	0.090[c]											
Physostigmine sulfate				0.074[c]											
Pilocarpine HCl			0.24	0.138[c]			0.22	0.38			4.08	0.22	0.52	89	4.0
Pilocarpine nitrate			0.23	0.132[c]			0.20	0.35			4.84	0.20	0.52	88	3.9
Piperocaine HCl				0.12[d]							5.22			65	5.7

Polyethylene glycol 300	0.12	0.034	0.12	0.069	0.12	0.141	0.12	0.216	0.13	0.378	6.73	0.13	0.52	53	3.8
Polyethylene glycol 400	0.08	0.022	0.08	0.047	0.09	0.098	0.09	0.153	0.09	0.272	8.50	0.11	0.52	0	4.4
Polyethylene glycol 1500	0.06	0.015	0.06	0.036	0.07	0.078	0.07	0.120	0.07	0.215	10.00	0.09	0.52	4	4.1
Polyethylene glycol 1540	0.02	0.005	0.02	0.012	0.02	0.028	0.03	0.047	0.03	0.094					
Polyethylene glycol 4000	0.02	0.004	0.02	0.008	0.02	0.02	0.020	0.033	0.02	0.067					
Polymyxin B sulfate	0.09		0.09	0.052			0.06	0.10	0.04	0.12					
Polysorbate 80	0.02	0.005	0.02	0.010	0.02	0.02	0.020	0.032	0.02	0.055					
Polyvinyl alcohol (99% hydrol)	0.02	0.004	0.02	0.008	0.02	0.020	0.02	0.035	0.03	0.075					
Polyvinylpyrrolidone	0.01	0.003	0.010	0.006	0.01	0.01	0.01	0.017	0.01	0.035					
Potassium acetate	0.59	0.172	0.59	0.342							1.53	0.59	0.52	0	7.6
Potassium chlorate											1.88			0	6.9
Potassium chloride			0.76	0.439[c]							1.19	0.76	0.52	0	5.9
Potassium iodide			0.34	0.196[c]							2.59	0.34	0.52	0	7.0
Potassium nitrate			0.56	0.324[c]							1.62	0.56	0	5.9	
Potassium phosphate			0.46	0.27							2.08	0.43	0.52	0	8.4
Potassium phosphate, monobasic			0.44	0.25							2.18	0.41	0.52	0	4.4
Potassium sulfate	0.44		0.44								2.11	0.43		0	6.6
Pralidoxime chloride	0.32	0.092	0.32	0.183	0.32	0.364					2.87	0.32	0.52	0	4.6
Prilocaine HCl	0.22	0.062	0.22	0.125	0.22	0.250	0.22	0.375			4.18	0.22	0.52	45	4.6
Procainamide HCl	0.22		0.22	0.13	0.19		0.19	0.33	0.17	0.49					
Procaine HCl	0.21		0.21	0.122[c]	0.19		0.19	0.33	0.18		5.05	0.18	0.52	91	5.6
Prochlorperazine edisylate	0.08	0.020	0.06	0.033	0.05	0.048	0.03	0.056	0.02	0.065					
Promazine HCl	0.18	0.050	0.13	0.077	0.09	0.102	0.07	0.112	0.05	0.137					

(continued)

Table 4.3 (continued)

	0.5 %		1 %		2 %		3 %		5 %		Iso-Osmotic Concentration[a]				
	E	D	E	D	E	D	E	D	E	D	%	E	D	H	pH
Proparacaine HCl	0.16	0.044	0.15	0.086	0.15	0.169	0.14	0.247	0.13	0.380	7.46	0.12	0.52		
Propiomazine HCl	0.18	0.050	0.15	0.084	0.12	0.133	0.10	0.165	0.08	0.215					
Propoxycaine HCl											6.40			16	5.3
Propylene glycol										0.17	2.00			100	5.5
Pyrathiazine HCl	0.22	0.065	0.17	0.095	0.11	0.123	0.08	0.140	0.06						
Pyridostigmine bromide	0.22	0.062	0.22	0.125	0.22	0.250	0.22	0.377			4.13	0.22	0.52	0	7.2
Pyridoxine HCl											3.05			31*	3.2
Quinacrine methanesulfonate				0.06[c]											
Quinine bisulfate			0.09	0.05			0.09	0.16							
Quinine dihydrochloride[a]			0.23	0.130[c]	0.19		0.19	0.33	0.18		5.07	0.18	0.52	trace*	2.5
Quinine hydrochloride			0.14	0.077[c]	0.11		0.11	0.19							
Quinine and urea HCl			0.23	0.13	0.21		0.21	0.36			4.50	0.20	0.52	64	2.9
Resorcinol		0.161[c]									3.30			96	5.0
Rolitetracycline	0.11	0.032	0.11	0.064	0.09	0.113	0.09	0.158	0.07	0.204					
Rose Bengal	0.08	0.02	0.07	0.04	0.07	0.083	0.07	0.124	0.07	0.198	14.9	0.06	0.52		
Rose Bengal B	0.08	0.022	0.08	0.044	0.08	0.087	0.08	0.131	0.08	0.218					
Scopolamine HBr			0.12	0.07	0.12		0.12	0.21	0.12	0.35	7.85	0.11	0.52	8	4.8
Scopolamine methylnitrate			0.16		0.14		0.14		0.13	6.95		0	6.0		
Secobarbital sodium			0.24	0.14	0.23		0.23	0.40			3.9	0.23	0.52	trace	9.8
Silver nitrate			0.33	0.190[c]							2.74	0.33	0.52	0*	5.0
Silver protein, mild			0.17	0.10	0.17		0.17	0.29	0.16	0.46	5.51	0.16	0.52	0	9.0

Silver protein, strong				0.06[d]											
Sodium acetate	0.24		0.46	0.267							2.0	0.45	0.52		
Sodium acetazolamide		0.068	0.23	0.135	0.23	0.271	0.23	0.406			3.85	0.23	0.52	0	7.3
Sodium aminosalicylate				0.170[c]							3.27	0.16		0	8.5
Sodium ampicillin	0.16	0.045	0.16	0.090	0.16	0.181	0.16	0.072	0.16	0.451	5.78		0.52	0	6.9
Sodium ascorbate											3.00			0	7.5
Sodium benzoate			0.40	0.230[c]							2.25	0.40	0.52	0	8.3
Sodium bicarbonate			0.65	0.375							1.39	0.65	0.52	0	4.1
Sodium biphosphate (H$_2$O)			0.40	0.23							2.45	0.37	0.52	0	4.0
Sodium biphosphate (2H$_2$O)			0.36								2.77	0.32		0	8.3
Sodium bismuth thioglycollate	0.20	0.055	0.19	0.107	0.18	0.208	0.18	0.303	0.17	0.493	5.29		0.52	0	3.0
Sodium bisulfite			0.61	0.35							1.5	0.61	0.52	0*	9.2
Sodium borate			0.42	0.241[c]							2.6	0.35	0.52	0	6.1
Sodium bromide			0.32				0.28				3.3	0.27		0	8.0
Sodium carbonate, monohydrated			0.60	0.346							1.56	0.58	0.52	100	11.1
Sodium cephalothin	0.18	0.05	0.17	0.095	0.16	0.179	0.15	0.259	0.14	0.400	6.80	0.13	0.52	partial	8.5
Sodium chloride			1.00	0.576[c]			1.00	1.73	1.00	2.88	0.9	1.00	0.52	0	6.7
Sodium citrate			0.31	0.178[c]			0.30	0.52			3.02	0.30	0.52	0	7.8
Sodium colistimethate	0.16	0.045	0.15	0.087	0.14	0.161	0.14	0.235	0.13	0.383	6.85	0.13	0.52	0	8.4
Sodium hypophosphite											1.60			0	7.3
Sodium iodide			0.39	0.222[c]							2.37	0.38	0.52	0	6.9
Sodium iodohippurate											5.92			0	7.3

(continued)

Table 4.3 (continued)

Substance	0.5 %		1 %		2 %		3 %		5 %		Iso-Osmotic Concentration[a]				
	E	D	E	D	E	D	E	D	E	D	%	E	D	H	pH
Sodium lactate	0.10	0.029	0.08	0.046	0.07	0.068	0.05	0.086			1.72			0	6.5
Sodium lauryl sulfate											5.30			0	8.4
Sodium mercaptomerin			0.67	0.386[c]							1.38	0.65	0.52	0	4.5
Sodium metabisulfite	0.18	0.050	0.18	0.099					0.15	0.445	6.00	0.15	0.52	5*	5.8
Sodium methicillin	0.14	0.039	0.14	0.078	0.16	0.192	0.16	0.281						0	
Sodium nafcillin					0.13	0.158	0.13	0.219	0.10	0.285				0	
Sodium nitrate			0.68								1.36	0.66		0	6.0
Sodium nitrite			0.84	0.480[c]							1.08	0.83		0*	8.5
Sodium oxacillin	0.18	0.050	0.17	0.095	0.15	0.177	0.15	0.257	0.14	0.408	6.64	0.14	0.52	0	6.0
Sodium phenylbutazone	0.19	0.054	0.18	0.104	0.17	0.202	0.17	0.298	0.17	0.488	5.34	0.17	0.52	0	
Sodium phosphate			0.29	0.168				0.47			3.33	0.27	0.52	0	9.2
Sodium phosphate, dibasic (2H$_2$O)			0.42	0.24							2.23	0.40	0.52	0	9.2
Sodium phosphate, dibasic (12H$_2$O)			0.22								4.45	0.20	0.52	0	9.2
Sodium propionate			0.61	0.35							1.47	0.61	0.52	0	7.8
Sodium salicylate			0.36	0.210[c]							2.53	0.36	0.52	0	6.7
Sodium succinate	0.32	0.092	0.32	0.184	0.31	0.361					2.90	0.31	0.52	0	8.5
Sodium sulfate, anhydrous			0.58	0.34							1.61	0.56	0.52	0	6.2
Sodium sulfite, exsiccated			0.65	0.38							1.45			0	9.6
Sodium sulfobromophthalein	0.07	0.019	0.06	0.034	0.05	0.060	0.05	0.084	0.04	0.123				0	
Sodium tartrate	0.33	0.098	0.33	0.193	0.33	0.385					2.72	0.33	0.52	0	7.3
Sodium thiosulfate			0.31	0.181[c]							2.98	0.30	0.52	0	7.4
Sodium warfarin	0.18	0.049	0.17	0.095	0.16	0.181	0.15	0.264	0.15	0.430	6.10	0.15	0.52	0	8.1
Sorbitol (Δ H$_2$O)											5.48			0	5.9

Sparteine sulfate	0.10	0.03	0.10	0.056	0.10	0.111	0.10	0.167	0.10	0.277	9.46	0.10	0.52	19*	3.5
Spectinomycin HCl	0.16	0.045	0.16	0.092	0.16	0.185	0.16	0.280	0.16	0.460	5.66	0.16	0.52	3	4.4
Streptomycin HCl			0.17	0.10[c]											
Streptomycin sulfate			0.07	0.036[c]			0.06	0.10	0.06	0.17					
Sucrose			0.08	0.047[c]			0.09	0.16	0.09	0.26	9.25	0.10	0.52	0	6.4
Sulfacetamide sodium			0.23	0.132[c]			0.23	0.40	0.23		3.85	0.23	0.52	0	8.7
Sulfadiazine sodium			0.24	0.14			0.24	0.38	0.21		4.24	0.21	0.52	0	9.5
Sulfamerazine sodium			0.23	0.13			0.21	0.36	0.21		4.53	0.20	0.52	0	9.8
Sulfapyridine sodium			0.23	0.13			0.21	0.36	0.21		4.55	0.20	0.52	5	10.4
Sulfathiazole sodium			0.22	0.13			0.20	0.35	0.20		4.82	0.19	0.52	0	9.9
Tartaric acid				0.143[c]						0.35	3.90			75*	1.7
Tetracaine HCl			0.18	0.109[c]			0.15	0.26	0.12						
Tetracycline HCl			0.14	0.081[c]		0.10									
Tetrahydrozoline HCl											4.10			60*	6.7
Theophylline				0.02*											
Theophylline sodium glycinate											2.94			0	8.9
Thiamine HCl				0.139[c]							4.24			87*	3.0
Thiethylperazine maleate	0.10	0.030	0.09	0.050	0.08	0.089	0.07	0.119	0.05	0.153					
Thiopental sodium				0.155[c]							3.50			7.4	10.3
Thiopropazate diHCl	0.20	0.053	0.16	0.090	0.12	0.137	0.10	0.170	0.08	0.222					
Thioridazine HCl	0.06	0.015	0.05	0.025	0.04	0.042	0.03	0.055	0.03	0.075					
Thiotepa	0.16	0.045	0.16	0.090	0.16	0.182	0.16	0.278	0.16	0.460	5.67	0.16	0.52	10*	8.2
Tridihexethyl chloride	0.16	0.047	0.16	0.096	0.16	0.191	0.16	0.28	0.16	0.463	5.62	0.16	0.52	97	5.4
Triethanolamine	0.20	0.058	0.21	0.121	0.22	0.252	0.22	0.383			4.05	0.22	0.52	100	10.7
Trifluoperazine 2HCl	0.18	0.052	0.18	0.100	0.13	0.144									
Triflupromazine HCl	0.10	0.031	0.09	0.051	0.05	0.061	0.04	0.073	0.03	0.092					

(continued)

Table 4.3 (continued)

Substance	0.5 %		1 %		2 %		3 %		5 %		Iso-Osmotic Concentration[a]				
	E	D	E	D	E	D	E	D	E	D	E	D	%	H	pH
Trimeprazine tartrate	0.10	0.023	0.06	0.035	0.04	0.045	0.03	0.052	0.02	0.061					
Trimethadione	0.23	0.069	0.23	0.133	0.22	0.257	0.22	0.378			0.21	0.52	4.22	100	6.0
Trimethobenzamide HCl	0.12	0.033	0.10	0.062	0.10	0.108	0.09	0.153	0.08	0.232					
Tripelennamine HCl				0.13[d]									5.50	100	6.3
Tromethamine	0.26	0.074	0.26	0.15	0.26	0.30	0.26	0.45			0.26	0.52	3.45	0	10.2
Tropicamide	0.10	0.03	0.09	0.050											
Trypan blue	0.26	0.075	0.26	0.150											
Tryparsamide				0.11[c]											
Tubocurarine chloride				0.076[c]											
Urea			0.59	0.34							0.55	0.52	1.63	100	6.6
Urethan				0.18[b]									2.93	100	6.3
Uridine	0.12	0.035	0.12	0.069	0.12	0.138	0.12	0.208	0.12	0.333	0.11	0.52	8.18	0*	6.1
Valethamate bromide	0.16	0.044	0.15	0.085	0.15	0.168	0.14	0.238	0.11	0.324					
Vancomycin sulfate	0.06	0.015	0.05	0.028	0.04	0.049	0.04	0.066	0.04	0.098					
Viomycin sulfate	0.08		0.08	0.05	0.07		0.07	0.12	0.07	0.20					
Xylometazoline HCl	0.22	0.065	0.21	0.121	0.20	0.232	0.20	0.342			0.19	0.52	4.68	88	5.0
Zinc phenolsulfonate												0*	5.40		5.4
Zinc sulfate	0.15		0.15	0.086[c]	0.13		0.12	0.23	0.12	0.35	0.12	0.52	7.65		

E, Sodium chloride equivalents; D, freezing-point depression, °C; H, hemolysis, %, at the concentration that is iso-osmotic with 0.9% NaCl, based on freezing-point determination or equivalent test; pH, approximate pH of solution studied for hemolytic action; *, change in appearance of erythrocytes and/or solution; †, pH determined after addition of blood.

[a] The unmarked values were taken from Hammarlund et al. and Sapp et al.

[b] Adapted from Lund et al.

[c] Adapted from British Pharmaceutical Codex.

[d] Obtained from several sources.

Note: See also Budavari S, ed. *Merck Index*, 11th edn, Rahway, NJ: Merck, 1988: MISC 79–103.

This table allows for correction of calculations when preparing isotonic solutions, providing sodium chloride equivalent correction (*I*) values (listed as E) for solutions of 0.5%, 1%, 2%, 3%, and 5% concentrations, as well as iso-osmotic concentrations for the pure solute. Since isotonic sodium chloride is 0.9%, the column for '1%' is the closest standard we can use from this table. The 'D' columns are for calculations based on freezing point depression.

Key Point

Since electrolytes do not always completely dissociate, correction values should be used when making tonicity calculations in order to more correctly account for true resulting tonicity. One common correction approach is to use the sodium chloride equivalent method.

What is accomplished using the correction factors is represented in Table 4.4, where the four colligative properties are re-expressed, with the correction factor (i). The constants for all four of the colligative property equations, without van't Hoff corrections, in aqueous solutions are listed in Table 4.4.

Application of van't Hoff *i* values

Reprising the calculations above, solving for *x*, a 1.0 molal concentration of particles will depress the freezing point of water by 1.86°C (K_f). This is the 'impact' of 1 mole of particles on water's freezing point. '*x*' is the amount of a given substance, for 1000 mL of water (1 kg), for 0.52°C depression of water's freezing point. Solving '*x*' for sodium chloride (two particles per dissociation, and so two moles of particles resulting from 1 mole of sodium chloride) gives us *x* = 8.17g sodium chloride for 1000 mL water. However, the question asks for the amount of solute required for 100 mL, which is 0.817g sodium chloride. This calculation is based on the assumption that sodium chloride completely dissociates in solution. What we are assuming is: 1 mole of sodium chloride provides 1.0 mole Na^+ + 1.0 mole Cl^-. So, 1 mole of sodium chloride provides 1.0 + 1.0 = 2.0 moles of particles. This enters into our calculation:

$$\frac{\text{MW of 1 mole of particles}}{1.86°C} = \frac{x}{0.52°C}; \quad \frac{\dfrac{58.5g}{2 \text{ moles of particles}}}{1.86°C} = \frac{x}{0.52°C}$$

$x = 0.817$ g NaCl (based on 100% dissociation).

Table 4.4 Constants for the four colligative properties for aqueous solutions		
Colligative property	**Proportionality constant in aqueous solution (assume 25°C), per molal**	**Unit**
Vapor pressure lowering	$*0.018p_1 = 0.43$	mmHg
Boiling point elevation	$K_b = 0.51$	Degrees per molal
Freezing point depression	$K_f = 1.86$	Degrees per molal
Osmotic pressure	$RT = 24.4$	Atmospheres (atm)

*0.018 is derived from: $X_B = \dfrac{(P_A^0 - P_A)}{(P_A^0)} = \dfrac{\dfrac{w_B}{M_B}}{\dfrac{1000}{M_B}} = \dfrac{m}{55.5} = 0.018\,m$

Now, the effects of incomplete dissociation, as studied by van't Hoff and others, become important. It is commonly understood that a 0.9% sodium chloride solution is 'isotonic' to human physiologic fluids. This solution, under the assumption of complete dissociation would be 0.9 g sodium chloride/100 mL solution. The molecular weight (MW) of sodium chloride is 58.44 g/mol. Through the above calculation, it is implied that an isotonic solution of sodium chloride would be 0.818g/100 mL, meaning an isotonic sodium chloride solution would be 0.82% – which is incorrect. Why is this? It is the effect the presence of ion pairs has on the assumptions, leading to an overestimation of the number of particles (and so tonicity) in the solution.

If, as van't Hoff suggested, we now assume only 80% dissociation of sodium chloride, this changes the collection of contributing moieties; 1 mole of sodium chloride provides 0.8 mole Na^+ + 0.8 mole Cl^-, but also 0.2 mole $\{Na+....Cl^-\}$ (the ion pair). So, 1 mole of sodium chloride provides 0.8 + 0.8 + 0.2 = 1.8 moles of particles – not 2:

$$1NaCl \rightarrow 0.8\,Na^+ + 0.8\,Cl^- + 0.2\{Na^+ ... Cl^-\} = 1.8 \text{ moles of particles}$$

(as previously illustrated in Figure 4.1).

Using the corrected values, the observed (accepted) amount of sodium chloride can now be confirmed:

$$\frac{MW \text{ of } 1 \text{ mole of particles}}{1.86°C} = \frac{x}{0.52°C}; \frac{\frac{58.5g}{1.8 \text{ moles of particles}}}{1.86°C} = \frac{x}{0.52°C}$$

1.8 moles particles = 0.8 + 0.8 + 0.2

$x = 0.909$ g NaCl (based on 80% dissociation).

The adjusted calculation now agrees much more closely with observed phenomena. The adjusted calculation implies 0.91% sodium chloride is isotonic, which is much more accurate – and the reason 'normal saline' is 0.9%, not 0.8%. How can the correction for incomplete dissociation be applied to our freezing point formula? By using the van't Hoff i values provided (fortunately) in tables such as Table 4.3. van't Hoff originally added the i value as a correction factor to the Morse equation for the osmotic pressure of dilute solutions of electrolytes, making the adjusted equation $\Pi = iRTc$, where c = molar concentration, rather than the molal concentration of the Morse equation. Since all of the colligative properties are related, they all can be expressed with this modification. For

Table 4.5	van't Hoff adjustments for the four colligative properties for aqueous solutions	
Colligative property	**Equation**	
Vapor pressure lowering	$\Delta P = 0.018 i P_r m$	
Boiling point elevation	$\Delta T_b = i K_b m$	
Freezing point depression	$\Delta T_f = i K_f m$	
Osmotic pressure (elevation)	$\Pi = i R T m$	

dilute solutions of electrolytes, the modified equations become those shown in Table 4.5.

Using these values from Table 4.4, inserted into the equations listed in Table 4.5, more accurate 'real-life' values of freezing point depression can be calculated. But why is this important? Because any of the four colligative properties could be used to measure the effect a solute has on the solution. Freezing point depression is easily measured, and there is an abundance of data with which two solutions might be compared. The goal of calculating a colligative effect is to try to match the magnitude of a colligative effect observed in physiologic solutions. The reason it is important that pharmaceutical solutions be physiologically equivalent actually is more directly related to osmotic pressure, but we use freezing point to indirectly calculate the osmotic effects of our solutions. By doing so, we ensure isotonicity of our solutions. The isotonicity depends on both osmotic pressure, and the mechanism by which it can be altered, diffusion.

Diffusion

Another important property of solutions and particles in solvents, though not considered a colligative property, is the property of diffusion from a region of higher concentration to one of lower concentration. Diffusion is the movement of molecules in liquids, the ease with which molecules diffuse across a membrane, and can be measured.

Molecules move down a concentration gradient at a rate proportional to the difference between the two concentrations, represented as C_1 and C_2, and inversely proportional to the distance over which the concentration change occurs $(x_1 - x_2)$, such that the movement is described by:

$$\frac{dC}{dx}$$

which represents the concentration gradient.

Diffusion modeling

Diffusion can be modeled using two mathematical descriptions: Fick's law of diffusion, and the Stokes–Einstein equation (Chapter 3, and below). Fick's law of diffusion is:

$$J = \frac{dM}{Sdt}$$

where J is the flux. Flux (J, g or moles/cm^2·sec) is a measure of the amount material (dM, g or moles), that crosses a defined area (S, cm^2), during a defined time (dt, seconds). So the flux equation provides a rate that particles move along the gradient. And therefore, J is proportional to the concentration gradient, dC/dx, where dC/dx is the change in concentration over (infinitely) small distances.

It is observed that flux is proportional to R and T, and inversely proportional to η, r, and N, as described below. Collectively, these are components of a diffusion coefficient, D, the Stokes–Einstein constant, as mentioned previously. D then, is dependent on the nature of the solvent and environmental conditions. D is described by the Stokes–Einstein equation:

$$D = \frac{RT}{6\pi\eta rN}$$

where D = diffusion coefficient (cm^2/s), R = molar gas constant, T = absolute temperature, η = viscosity of the solvent, r = radius of (an assumed spherical) particle and N = Avogadro's number.

Substituting the concentration gradient, dC/dx and D into Fick's law gives:

$$J = -D\frac{dC}{dx}$$

where dC = change in concentration and dx = distance (change) from the particle surface.

When the equations for Fick's law and the Stokes–Einstein equation are combined, this gives:

$$-\frac{dM}{dt} = DA\left(\frac{dc}{dx}\right)$$

where M = grams or moles, and is expressed in negative terms, as a loss of material, and dM/dt = the amount of substance diffusing over time across a plane of surface A.

Together, the Morse equation, Fick's law, and the Stokes–Einstein equation tell us that 1) diffusion is related to surface area and thickness of the membrane, and to the concentration gradient, and 2) diffusion is related to particle size, solution viscosity and temperature of the medium. Diffusion has direct implications on the compatibility of pharmaceutical preparations with biological systems.

Key Point

Diffusion of solutes and dispersed particles affects compatibility of drug delivery systems with the body, and is related to:

- Surface area
- Membrane thickness
- Concentration gradient

Applications to dosage form preparation

Why are diffusion and colligative properties important for pharmaceutical and biological systems? It is because of the relatively specific tolerance for solute concentrations by tissues. We need to make preparations that are isotonic or isosmotic (in general, for physiologic systems, the two are synonymous), and it is diffusion that alters osmotic pressure – and tonicity – in physiologic systems. Still, why is isotonicity important? It is because, resilient as biological systems are, there are limits to solute gradients and tonicity beyond which damage will occur. Therefore, when preparing solutions for use in the body, there are limits, both lower and higher, to the number of particles that can be contained in the preparations, per unit volume. The strictness of the range varies somewhat, depending on the tissue. Recall that, through a semipermeable (i.e., 'biological') membrane, water will tend to move to balance concentrations – or osmotic pressures – on both sides of the membrane. Even though we account for ions or particles, it is the movement of water with which we are ultimately concerned. As stated previously, osmotic pressure (Π) of a solution can be roughly described by the Morse equation. Since it has been explained that the van't Hoff modification to the Morse factor lends more accuracy to calculations, in practice we rarely need to perform calculations with the Morse equation, but we do need to ensure the molal concentrations of solutes 'add up' properly. To keep the illustrations simple, we will temporarily assume pharmaceutical solutions behave ideally. Thus, within fairly strict parameters, we need the osmotic pressure, Π, on each side of a membrane to be nearly identical. If this is accomplished, there is no tendency for either side of the membrane (most notably enclosed areas, such as red blood cells) to expand or contract as a result of osmotic pressure differences from one side to the other. Examples of when this is not achieved are rather dire (Figure 4.2).

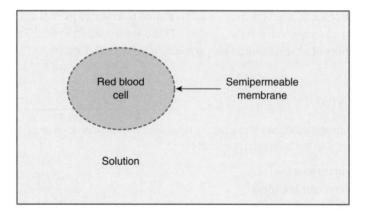

Figure 4.2 Osmotic pressure and biological membranes

There are many biological membranes in the body. Some of them (e.g., erythrocytes) are extremely sensitive to osmotic pressure that is either too high or too low. In cases where osmotic pressure of biological fluids – or pharmaceuticals – create too low or high osmotic pressure, damage can occur to tissues.

If the osmotic pressure outside the red blood cell is greater than that inside, water will tend to move out of the cell, shrinking it, and ultimately cause crenation. Again, for osmotic pressure, it is the movement of water, not ions or particles, with which we are concerned. If the opposite conditions are true, water will move into the cell, expanding it and ultimately cause lysis. Other types of tissue (other than cells) can also be prone to negative consequences occurring as a result of improper balancing of osmotic pressures. The magnitude of osmotic pressure causes a 'tone' in biological membranes, and so osmotic pressure and tonicity are considered synonymous. In practice, there are some occasions when it is actually our intention to make something hypertonic or hypotonic, in order to achieve a goal related to the resulting osmotic imbalance. But, most times we wish to keep our preparations at 'biological' tonicity, meaning isotonic.

Our objective then, especially for parenteral solutions, is to make them isotonic with respect to physiological fluids. Based on colligative behavior, we can determine the concentration of solute necessary to make a solution iso-osmotic with physiological fluids. And, as previously stated, iso-osmotic solutions generally are isotonic. Also mentioned previously, it is known that 0.280 moles of particles per liter = concentration of particles in physiological fluids. Using the Morse equation, it can be calculated that $\Pi = 0.082 \times 310 \times 0.280 = 7.12$ atm (where $R = 0.082$, and $T =$ normal body temperature $= 37°C = 311$ kelvin, and 0.280 M is considered isotonic). 0.280 M is our target if using osmotic pressure to calculate isotonicity.

As stated previously, any of the colligative properties could be used to calculate the necessary ingredient concentrations to make isotonic preparations using the formulae for the particular colligative property. However, in practice, the most common methods utilize standardizing either via freezing point depression (discussed above) using the sodium chloride equivalent method, or a streamlined method. The sodium chloride equivalent method is really what the previous discussion has presented: setting sodium chloride as a known entity, with regard to its effects on freezing point depression, then using a 'calibration' number to make other useful solutes 'equivalent' to a known amount of sodium chloride in their freezing point depression actions. An example of the sodium chloride equivalent method, used in a practical way, is presented in the following example:

Rx   Ephedrine sulfate   25 mg/mL
           Make isotonic with boric acid
           Sterile Water for Injection qs ad   15 mL

a) From Table 4.3, the sodium chloride equivalent of a 1% (1 g/100 mL) solution of ephedrine sulfate is 0.13°.

b) This prescription is for 25 mg/mL = 2500 mg/100 mL = 2.5 g/100 mL = 2.5% solution.

c) Calculating the freezing point depression for this concentration of ephedrine sulfate is approximately:

$$\frac{1\%}{0.13} = \frac{2.5\%}{x}$$

$$x = 0.33°.$$

d) Subtract this from the target freezing point depression of −0.52°.

0.52 − 0.33 = 0.19°. This is the amount still needed to make the solution isotonic, as measured by freezing point depression, according to sodium chloride equivalents.

e) The prescription calls for boric acid to be used as a tonicity adjusting agent. Referring to our reference table (Table 4.3), the freezing point depression, as calculated via sodium chloride equivalents, of a 1% boric acid solution is 0.29°.

f) Calculate the concentration of boric acid that is needed to provide the additional freezing point depression (via sodium chloride equivalents) required:

$$\frac{1\%}{0.29} = \frac{x\%}{0.19 \text{ required}}$$

$$x = 0.66\%.$$

g) Calculate the weight of boric acid in 15 mL of 0.66% solution:
0.66% × 15 mL = 0.0990 g = 99.0 mg.

USP (White–Vincent) method

It is easy to see that, though the sodium chloride equivalent method provides reliable conversions, another, potentially simpler, method might be preferred. To determine how much of a tonicity-adjusting agent is needed to render a drug solution isotonic, a simplified freezing point method is called the USP Method, or White–Vincent Method, with the equation:

$$V = w \times E \times 111.1$$

where V = volume (mL) of 100 mL isotonic solution that may be made simply with the drug and water

w = weight (g) of the drug

E = the drug's sodium chloride equivalent

111.1 = volume (mL) of the solution resulting from a 0.9% sodium chloride solution.

This is from:

$$\frac{0.9\,\text{g NaCl}}{100\,\text{mL isotonic solution}} = \frac{1\,\text{g NaCl}}{x\,\text{mL isotonic solution}}; x = 111.1\,\text{mL}$$

This is then set up as:

$$111.1 \times \left(\text{drug's } E \text{ value}\right) \times (\text{g of drug})$$

To utilize this method, isotonicity values, listed as V values must be known. Table 4.6 lists V values for some common solutes.

Key Point

For purposes of USP (White–Vincent) tonicity calculations, a good number to remember is that 111.1 mL is the isotonic volume that results from adding sodium chloride to 100 mL of water.

An example of the USP (White–Vincent) method is as follows:

Rx	NaI	2%
	Make isotonic	
	Purified Water qs ad	15 mL

The V value for NaI is 13.0; the E value is 0.39.

a) g of drug in solution: (2 g/100 mL) × 15 mL = 0.30 g;

b) V value of NaI = 13.0 mL water needed to make isotonic.

Or, $V = w \times E \times 111.1$: $V = (0.30\text{ g NaI})(0.39\text{ g NaCl}/1\text{ g NaI})(111.1\text{ mL isotonic solution}/1\text{ g NaCl}) = 13.0\text{ mL water made isotonic with NaI only.}$

So, 2.0 mL must be made isotonic with NaCl; 0.9 g/100 mL × 2.0 mL = 0.018 g NaCl. Therefore, 0.018 g NaCl and 2.0 mL water need to be added.

Table 4.6 Isotonic solution V values

Drug (0.3 g)	Water Needed for Isotonicity (mL)	Drug (0.3 g)	Water Needed for Isotonicity (mL)	Drug (0.3 g)	Water Needed for Isotonicity (mL)
Alcohol	21.7	Epinephrine bitartrate	6.0	Potassium chloride	25.3
Ammonium chloride	37.3	Epinephrine hydrochloride	9.7	Silver nitrate	11.0
Amobarbital sodium	8.3	Ethylmorphine hydrochloride	5.3	Silver protein, mild	5.7
Amphetamine phosphate	11.3	Fluorescein sodium	10.3	Sodium acetate	15.3
Amphetamine sulfate	7.3	Glycerin	11.7	Sodium bicarbonate	21.7
Antipyrine	5.7	Holocaine hydrochloride	6.7	Sodium biphosphate, anhydrous	15.3
Apomorphine hydrochloride	4.7	Homatropine hydrobromide	5.7	Sodium biphosphate	13.3
Ascorbic acid	6.0	Homatropine methylbromide	6.3	Sodium bisulfite	20.3
Atropine methylbromide	4.7	Hyoscyamine sulfate	4.7	Sodium borate	14.0
Atropine sulfate	4.3	Neomycin sulfate	3.7	Sodium iodide	13.0
Bacitracin	1.7	Oxytetracycline hydrochloride	4.3	Sodium metabisulfite	22.3
Barbital sodium	10.0	Penicillin G, potassium	6.0	Sodium nitrate	22.7
Bismuth potassium tartrate	3.0	Penicillin G, sodium	6.0	Sodium phosphate	9.7
Boric acid	16.7	Pentobarbital sodium	8.3	Sodium propionate	20.3
Butacaine sulfate	6.7	Phenobarbital sodium	8.0	Sodium sulfite, exsiccated	21.7
Caffeine and sodium benzoate	8.7	Physostigmine salicylate	5.3	Sodium thiosulfate	10.3
Calcium chloride	17.0	Pilocarpine hydrochloride	8.0	Streptomycin sulfate	2.3
Calcium chloride ($6H_2O$)	11.7	Pilocarpine nitrate	7.7	Sulfacetamide sodium	7.7
Chlorobutanol (hydrated)	8.0	Piperocaine hydrochloride	7.0	Sulfadiazine sodium	8.0
Chlortetracycline sulfate	4.3	Polymyxin B sulfate	3.0	Sulfamerazine sodium	7.7

(continued)

Table 4.6 *(continued)*

Drug (0.3 g)	Water Needed for Isotonicity (mL)	Drug (0.3 g)	Water Needed for Isotonicity (mL)	Drug (0.3 g)	Water Needed for Isotonicity (mL)
Cocaine hydrochloride	5.3	Potassium nitrate	18.7	Sulfapyridine sodium	7.7
Cupric sulfate	6.0	Potassium phosphate, monobasic	14.7	Sulfathiazole sodium	7.3
Dextrose, anhydrous	6.0	Procainamide hydrochloride	7.3	Tetracaine hydrochloride	6.0
Dibucaine hydrochloride	4.3	Procaine hydrochloride	7.0	Tetracycline hydrochloride	4.7
Dihydrostreptomycin sulfate	2.0	Scopolamine hydrobromide	4.0	Viomycin sulfate	2.7
Ephedrine hydrochloride	10.0	Scopolamine methylnitrate	5.3	Zinc chloride	20.3
Ephedrine sulfate	7.7	Secobarbital sodium	8.0	Zinc sulfate	5.0

[a] This table of isotonic solution values shows volumes in mL of water to be added to 300 mg of the specified drug in sterile water to produce an isotonic solution. The addition of an isotonic vehicle (commonly referred to as diluting solution) to make 30 mL yields a 1% solution. Solutions prepared as directed above are iso-osmotic with 0.9% sodium chloride solution but may not be isotonic with blood (see Table 4.3 for hemolysis data).

[b] The V values for drugs that do not appear in Table 4.6 but are listed in Table 4.3 can be calculated from the sodium chloride equivalent for 1% drug. *Example*—Calculate the V value for anileridine HCl (Table 4.3 defines $E = 0.19$).

$$\frac{100\text{ml Soln}}{0.9\text{ NaCl}} \times \frac{0.19\text{g Nacl}}{1\text{ g drug}} \times 0.3\text{ g drug} = 6.33\text{ mL Soln}$$

for dilute solution

6.33 mL soln $\cong 6.33$ mL water $\therefore V = 6.33$ mL water/0.3 g drug.

Summary

In summary, the four colligative properties of solutions can be used to prepare solutions that are isotonic, and thus physiologically compatible. Care must be exercised that deviation from 'ideal' solutions is a universal phenomenon, and that calculations should take into account divergence from ideality. Understanding diffusion properties of liquids as well as the colligative properties of solutions helps in the thoughtful preparation of isotonic solutions for drug delivery systems.

Self-assessment questions

1. What does colligative mean? What is a colligative property?

2. What are the four colligative properties? What are the equations that are used to express them?

3. Why do we need correction values, such as van't Hoff *i* values, for calculating colligative effects on dilute solutions?

4. What are some potential consequences of ignoring colligative properties when preparing drug delivery systems?

5. What does isotonic mean?

6. How is diffusion related to tonicity?

7. What parameters of diffusion affect tonicity? Can we control any of these parameters?

8. Why do you think both isotonicity calculation methods discussed are based on sodium chloride?

9. A prescription asks for 500 mL of a 1% aqueous sodium salicylate solution. Use the sodium chloride equivalents method to calculate how many grams of sodium chloride are needed to make this isotonic. The sodium chloride equivalent for sodium salicylate is 0.36.

10. A preparation calls for 15 mL of a 3% ephedrine hydrochloride solution. Use the USP method to calculate how to make this isotonic. The *E* value for ephedrine hydrochloride = 0.30; the *V* value = 10.0 mL.

5

Interfacial phenomena

Learning objectives

Upon completion of this chapter, you should be able to answer the following questions:

- What is a surface?
- What is an interface?
- How do surfaces and interfaces differ?
- What are surface tension and interfacial tension?
- Why do liquids tend to form spheres?
- Why is it sometimes useful to decrease surface or interfacial tension?
- What is a surfactant, and how do surfactants work?
- Describe the relationship between the hydrophilic lipophilic balance number of a surfactant, and its usefulness for decreasing surface/interfacial tension between two phases.

Many drug delivery systems rely on interfacial properties to function properly. Interfacial properties are those occurring between two phases (gas, liquid, solid) between a phase and 'air', or for thermodynamic considerations within portions of the same phase. The latter is more applicable to 'thought' experiments or questions when considering internal interactions for comparison or calculation. As always, intermolecular interactions are central to the observed phenomena at interfaces.

Interfaces

What are interfaces? Interfaces are the boundaries where two different phases meet and from which each may be distinguished – beginning and ending points. Interfacial properties dictate how well, if at all, two phases may interact. As discussed in Chapter 3, they are important when considering liquid spreading and wetting of solids. Interfaces occur between liquids and gasses, liquids and liquids, and between liquids and solids. Since liquid drug delivery systems are extremely

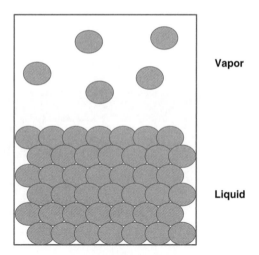

Figure 5.1 A simple interaction between a liquid and vapor or air

A pure liquid in a container (such as a beaker) with a vapor phase above the bulk liquid.

common, liquid–liquid interfaces will be the form most emphasized in this discussion. When speaking of liquid–liquid systems, a good example can be oil and water (or perhaps oil and vinegar, such as salad dressing). These two liquids are immiscible, normally remaining as two distinct liquid phases, and definitely forming no solution. First, a closer look at interfaces.

A simple form of interface is that between a liquid in a beaker and the environment above it (vapor or 'air'; Figure 5.1). This type of interface is more often referred to as a surface, as the vapor phase many times is not an important consideration, since these are molecules in the air above the liquid, which originate in the bulk. In this example, it can be imagined there will be a lack of symmetry of forces when the two phases meet: the liquid is more dense than the vapor, and is dominated by potential energy of attraction. The forces will be illustrated below. Strong intermolecular interactions keep the liquid in a predominantly condensed state, and potential energy dominates here. Kinetic energy is the dominant force in the vapor phase, where macroscopic actions have their origins in molecular actions.

Between a liquid and its vapor phases is a surface, which is not a true 'interface' as the vapor is impure, and the condensed phase is in contact with a vapor. Correctly speaking, the liquid has a surface. The surface of the bulk liquid is in equilibrium with the vapor. If observed from above, the bulk liquid would appear to be a flat, quiescent layer of liquid and have a reasonably definite boundary. One cannot observe the surface of the vapor. Therefore, in this simplest of examples, it must be pointed out that a condensed phase (solid or liquid) in association with a gas will have a surface as opposed to an interface (Figure 5.2). However, many actions that occur at a surface are applicable to interfaces.

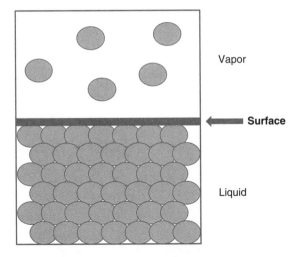

Figure 5.2 Between a condensed phase and a vapor phase is a surface

Between a condensed phase (solid or liquid) and its associated vapor phase is a surface – analogous to, but distinct from, an interface.

A more general term that can be applied to this situation is an interfacial region (Figure 5.3). This term implies a gradual transition between the two phases, whereas the term interface describes a more abrupt delineation. 'Region' allows for a changeover between two phases, while the term 'interface' describes a demarcation. The term 'interfacial region' can be used to recognize the distinction

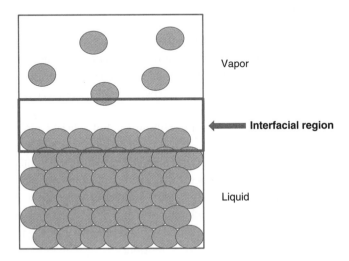

Figure 5.3 Interfacial region between condensed and vapor phases

For a simple condensed phase-vapor phase system, 'interfacial region' is a better descriptor than 'surface' or 'interface.' However, the three terms are often considered synonymous in practice.

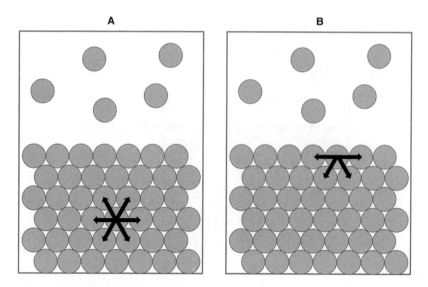

Figure 5.4 Asymmetrical forces exist in the interfacial region

Molecules in bulk (A) are exposed to symmetrical forces from surrounding molecules, while molecules in the interface (B) are pulled into the bulk, minimizing the interfacial area. Both of these should be imagined to be in three dimensions.

from a true interface, while allowing treatment of surfaces in a similar fashion to interfaces.

Interfacial forces and surface tension

Returning to the asymmetry of forces acting at a surface, it can be illustrated that molecules within the bulk have different molecular interactions than those at the surface. Within the bulk, the interactions tend to cancel each other, resulting in no net force, or symmetrical forces. This is not the case in the interfacial region where forces are not symmetrical (Figure 5.4).

The vapor molecules do exert some pull on the bulk surface molecules, but since the vapor molecules are relatively dilute, their forces on the more densely packed bulk molecules are minimal. The result is that there is a net pull on surface molecules into the bulk. This pull is the cause of the phenomenon observed that liquids reduce their surface area, reducing the number of molecules at the surface as much as possible. The inward pull and reduction of exposed molecules at the surface creates a curved surface (a meniscus) that is often visible. The force that is manifest via the meniscus is called surface tension.

In order to force the surface of a liquid to increase its surface area, in effect, the edges would need to be 'pulled' outward (which, it may be noted, cannot be achieved with a solid; Figure 5.5). To accomplish this pull, work must be done to

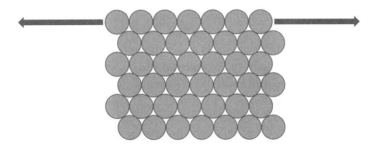

Figure 5.5 Expansion of the liquid interface

In order to oppose unbalanced forces that naturally cause the surface of a liquid to contract and curve, work has to be done against this force.

overcome the thermodynamic tendency of the liquid to minimize the exposed liquid surface.

As the surface area is expanded, molecules from the bulk flow up, into the interface, and so the number of molecules at the surface increases. Work against the pull of the bulk must be done to move the molecules to the surface and enlarge the surface area. Recall that free energy (ΔG) is the useful, purposeful energy that can be either obtained from a spontaneous process or that has to be put into a process that is not spontaneous. Since increasing the surface area of the example liquid is not spontaneous, to accomplish this, the Gibbs free energy change (ΔG) that is associated with this work is positive (work input is needed). That is, increasing the surface area(s) of a liquid increases the free energy (ΔG) of the system as a whole. This work done is against the opposing surface tension (γ) of the liquid. Surface tension is created by the asymmetrical inward pull by the bulk. The amount of work (W) done is proportional to the change in the liquid's surface area (ΔA). This can be represented by the following equation:

$$W = \Delta G = \gamma \Delta A.$$

Of interest is the surface tension, γ. So, rearranging the equation provides:

$$\gamma = \frac{\Delta G}{\Delta A}$$

where

W = work (J)
ΔG = Gibbs free energy change (J)
γ = proportionality constant = surface or interfacial tension (J/m²)
ΔA = change in surface area (m²).

γ is a proportionality constant for the comparison of system free energy and surface area changes. More than that, γ provides a means of gauging what needs to be accomplished in order to cause the changes in G or A to occur, as increasing surface area is a prerequisite to wetting of solids and imparting solubilities to otherwise immiscible materials. It can be noted that γ is a two-dimensional value (i.e., J/m^2), rather than three-dimensional (i.e., m^3). When using ergs, the units may appear one-dimensional! An erg (dynes × cm) is a force exerted over a distance, meaning γ (dynes/cm) is a force per unit of distance (two-dimensional); ergs/cm^2 is the same as dynes/cm and γ is energy (ergs or J/m^2) that acts parallel to the surface. In order to increase surface area, work must be done against γ. For water, the work that must be done to overcome surface tension (γ) can be expressed as either 73 ergs/cm^2 or 73 dynes/cm (only the units change). Often there arises a need to decrease surface tension (e.g., to improve wetting of a solid by a liquid). In order to decrease the surface tension of a liquid in contact with air, a surface active agent (surfactant) can be employed, as surfactants decrease γ. Surfactants are substances that adsorb at interfaces, decreasing surface tensions between liquids and air, liquids and solids, and between differing liquids. They do so by virtue of being amphiphilic in nature. They decrease contact angles for solids, facilitating wetting and dissolution, and allow dissimilar liquids to mix – not as solutions, but as dispersions.

Interfacial tension

So far, the condition when a liquid is in contact with its vapor phase has been described, and it has been shown that a surface is present between the two phases. A more complex system involves two immiscible liquids, such as oil and water rather than a liquid and vapor. In this situation, the two liquids will share an interface, rather than a surface. An interface involves more interactions outside of the bulk than occur at a surface (Figure 5.6). In this situation, an interfacial tension rather than a surface tension is present. However, overcoming interfacial tension is analogous to that of surface tension, only the aim is to promote mixing of the two liquids.

When two liquids are in contact, the molecules are distinctly different, but weak (intermolecular) interactions can occur across the interface (i.e., London dispersion forces). So molecules are still pulled into the respective bulk liquids because of lack of symmetry with regard to the forces across the interface of each liquid. This is analogous to interactions between a vapor and a liquid surface, only the pull into the bulk is not as unbalanced as when vapor is the second 'phase.' Though the interactions across the liquid–liquid interface are weak, the result is a diminished pull of interfacial molecules into their respective bulk phases. In order to facilitate these interactions, and perhaps induce mixing of otherwise immiscible liquids, as for surface tension, a surfactant can be employed to effect interfacial tension. Surfactants can impact the actions of liquids at interfaces more than at surfaces. Surfactant agents lower surface tension. They also decrease interfacial

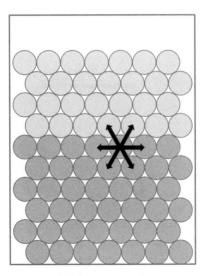

Figure 5.6 Molecular forces in the liquid–liquid interface

Force interactions across a liquid–liquid interface are possible. The higher density of the neighboring liquid phase means molecules are close enough to interact. This results in a diminished pull of interfacial molecules into the bulk of each phase, compared to when only vapor is in contact with a liquid bulk. The two liquids share an interface, rather than a surface.

tension along a liquid surface, between two liquids, but how? Many surfactant molecules are amphiphilic, and so possess some degree of solubility both in oil and water. Recall that amphiphiles are molecules that have both polar and nonpolar regions. The nonpolar region(s) contain hydrocarbon chains. The difference in electronegativity (a means of quantifying the predisposition of an atom to attract electrons) between hydrogen (2.2) and carbon (2.6) is negligible, so there is no large net 'pull' in this type of region. The polar region(s) contain groups such as hydroxyls, esters and aldehydes that can be ionic, charged regions. The degree of solubility in each type of liquid depends on the relative proportions of hydrophilic and hydrophobic regions. Ultimately, amphiphiles orient in such a way as to minimize the free energy of the whole system.

It was earlier discussed that intermolecular interactions cause liquids to attract into their respective bulks. If two liquids come in contact and possess similar intermolecular interaction types, they will be more predisposed to mixing than those possessing dissimilar forces. An oil utilizes only weak, London-type forces of attraction between its molecules, whereas water uses dipoles, hydrogen bonds and other strong forces between its molecules. This disparity would lead to the (correct) assumption that oil and water would be unlikely to mix. In addition, oil is less dense than water or vinegar, and so will rise to the top of the two liquids. If work is applied in the form of agitation (stirring), the two surface tensions are overcome, the two surface areas are expanded, both liquids are distributed, and water and oil will temporarily disperse in one another (Figure 5.7). In order

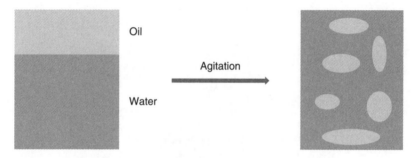

Figure 5.7 Agitation of oil and water

Agitation temporarily distributes the oil throughout the water.

to maintain this mixture, work must be continuously applied because, though dispersed, the condition is energetically unfavorable for both liquids.

When agitation is stopped, the natural tendency of the system is to reduce its interfacial free energy, so each liquid will move to assume more energetically favorable conditions. As discussed in Chapters 3 and 7, the dispersed liquid (in this example, oil) will naturally form spheres, which is the most efficient geometric conformation, to decrease the interfacial area between the two liquids. Eventually the spherical oil droplets will coalesce and rise to the surface of the water, and the original, more energetically favorable condition will be reassumed: the oil will sit on top of the water.

Making stability from instability

For various reasons, many drug delivery systems require oils and aqueous solutions to be mixed – or dispersed – in one another because use of a solution dosage form is not an option (Chapter 6 and 7). Therefore, methods must be employed that will enable a fundamentally unstable system to be at least temporarily stabilized, in order for the dosage form to be prepared and delivered to the patient. For most common pharmaceutical uses this means stabilizing the dispersion of an oil in water, though there are some systems that require an aqueous phase to be dispersed in an oil. For either situation, decreasing the free energy of liquids, by reducing interfacial tension, is the foundation for success. First, the discussion regarding work of adhesion and cohesion, and surface tension, introduced in Chapter 3, will be expounded upon.

Adhesion and cohesion – Two dissimilar liquids

The discussion in Chapter 3 was in regard to the work and energy requirements of the wetting of a solid with a liquid, as an initial step toward dissolution of the solid in the liquid. When the actions between a liquid and solid were illustrated, the two components – or phases – involved included a solid and a liquid, and the work of adhesion (between molecules of the liquid and solid), and the work of cohesion (between molecules of the liquid) were differentiated. Of application to the topic of interfacial phenomena are the forces involved between two dissimilar liquids, oil and water. Analogous to the forces within and between a solid and liquid, those within and between oil and water are now the focus: the forces of adhesion and cohesion.

The work of adhesion is a more straightforward illustration than is the work of cohesion. This now is with regard to the work between two dissimilar liquids, L_1 and L_2, and an illustration much like that of Figure 3.13(A) can be used. With two dissimilar liquids, the interfacial tension can be denoted as γ_{L1L2}. The work required to separate the two liquids then is:

$$W_A = \gamma_{L1} + \gamma_{L2}$$

where

W_A = work of adhesion between liquids 1 and 2
γ_{L1} = surface tension of liquid 1
γ_{L2} = surface tension of liquid 2.

Within each liquid there also exist cohesive forces. These are more difficult to illustrate, but if a liquid can be imagined to have two 'halves' that are physically drawn away from each other, it can also be imagined there are cohesive forces, analogous to the adhesive forces between oil and water, that must be overcome, in order for these two 'halves' of a liquid to separate. The work of cohesion, as was discussed in Chapter 3 (Figure 3.13(B)), is:

$$W_C = \gamma_L + \gamma_L = 2\gamma_L$$

where

W_C = work of cohesion within ½ of a 'single liquid,'
γ_L = imaginary surface tension between two halves of a liquid.

As is sometimes true for wetting of solids by liquids, enabling oil and water to remain mixed requires a surfactant – an agent that decreases the surface tension of one, or both components, allowing work to be decreased ($W = \gamma\Delta A$). To disperse the oil in water, the oil's surface area must be increased, but not at the expense of (continuous) work. Empirically, it can be seen that if surface area increases, surface tension, γ, must decrease. This is exactly what surfactants do (decrease surface tension). When two liquids are in contact, it is the interfacial tension, rather than the surface tension, which is referred to. Surfactants, by virtue of their interactions with both liquids, enhance weak (London-type) interactions between water and oil, decrease the cohesive dominance within each liquid and impart a less 'heterophobic' character to both.

Surfactants in drug delivery systems

Application of surfactant theory to drug delivery systems is straightforward. In Chapter 3, the aim was the improved wetting and dissolution of solids by decreasing surface tension of the liquid. The goal was to facilitate dissolution. In the present discussion, the aim is to improve miscibility of two liquids by decreasing interfacial tension between the two liquids. The goal is to facilitate the mixing of liquids. Two liquids in a pharmaceutical preparation may not be immiscible, but they may not mix as quickly or completely as needed. Use of a surfactant can facilitate the mixing. In Chapter 7, the use of surfactants to help create emulsions (dispersions of at least two immiscible liquids) will be discussed. A method of quantifying the relative hydrophilicity (or hydrophobicity) of a surfactant can be helpful in choosing a surfactant most suitable for the dosage form requirements. One method is the hydrophilic lipophilic balance (HLB) numbering system, which provides an arbitrary scale (normally from 0 to 20) that represents the relative hydrophilicity of many surfactants. The higher the HLB, the more hydrophilic is the surfactant (Table 5.1). It is also important to have a guide as to what HLB is required for a given material, and its application (Table 5.2). Then, a surfactant best suited for the liquid(s) can be selected. Surfactants with differing HLB values often can be blended to provide a desired balance. Using guides such as those in Table 5.2, proper surfactants can be chosen that optimize the required characteristics of the delivery system.

Emulsions are discussed in Chapter 7. However, HLB has applications for both surfactants and emulsifying agents.

Table 5.1	A typical hydrophilic lipophilic balance numbering system	
HLB range	Use	High HLB = good **water** solubility
10–18	Solubilizers	
13–15	Detergents	
8–18	Oil-in-water emulsions	
7–9	Wetting agents	
4–6	Water-in-oil emulsions	Low HLB = good **oil** solubility

HLB = hydrophilic lipophilic balance.

Table 5.2 HLB values for some common emulsifiers		
Agent	**HLB**	**Class**
Oleic acid	1.0	Anionic
Ethylene glycol distearate	1.5	Nonionic
Sorbitan tristearate (Span 65)	2.1	Nonionic
Glyceryl monooleate	3.3	Nonionic
Propylene glycol monostearate	3.4	Nonionic
Glyceryl monostearate	3.8	Nonionic
Sorbitan monooleate (Span 80)	4.3	Nonionic
Sorbitan monostearate (Span 60)	4.7	Nonionic
Diethylene glycol monolaurate	6.1	Nonionic
Sorbitan monopalmitate (Span 40)	6.7	Nonionic
Acacia	8.0	Anionic
Polyoxyethylene lauryl ether (Brij 30)	9.7	Nonionic
Polyoxyethylene monostearate (Myrj 45)	11.1	Nonionic
Triethanolamine oleate	12.0	Anionic
Polyoxyethylene sorbitan monostearate (Tween 60)	14.9	Nonionic
Polyoxyethylene sorbitan monooleate (Tween 80)	15.0	Nonionic
Polyoxyethylene sorbitan monolaurate (Tween 20)	16.7	Nonionic
Pluronic F 68	17.0	Nonionic
Sodium oleate	18.0	Anionic
Potassium oleate	20.0	Anionic
Cetrimonium bromide	23.3	Cationic
Cetylpyridinium chloride	26.0	Cationic
Poloxamer 188	29.0	Nonionic
Sodium lauryl sulfate	40.0	Anionic

Summary

Control of the intermolecular interactions that occur between liquids, and between liquids and other phases, is important for creating drug delivery systems that require liquids to wet or mix with other components of the drug delivery system, that they are not naturally 'inclined to be with.' In order to cause liquids to act in these ways, manipulation of the surface or interfacial tensions is required. Surfactants are employed to change surface/interfacial tensions, decreasing the work required for mixing and wetting. Use of a system, such as the HLB ranking, enables thoughtful planning of drug delivery systems in which surface wetting, dissolution, and mixing of components is facilitated, more permanent, and more predictable.

Self-assessment questions

1. What is a surface?

2. What is an interface?

3. What are surface tension and interfacial tension?

4. Why is it sometimes useful to decrease surface or interfacial tension?

5. What is 'HLB,' and how is it useful?

6. Why do droplets form a spherical shape?

7. Why is the surface tension of water greater than the surface tension of oil?

8. Why is interfacial tension less than surface tension?

9. Why does a surfactant lower surface tension?

10. Two surfactants are employed in a drug delivery system. Surfactant 1 has a HLB of 6 and Surfactant 2 has a HLB of 8. If the two surfactants are compatible, and used in equal proportion, the resulting combination would be categorized for what use?

6

Disperse systems – Colloids

Learning objectives

Upon completion of this chapter, you should be able to answer the following questions:

- What is a dispersion?
- What are liquid colloids, or colloidal dispersions, and how do they differ from other liquid drug delivery systems?
- What is the approximate size of colloidal particles, and how does this differ from particle sizes of other liquid delivery systems?
- What characteristics make liquid colloidal dispersions unique from other liquid delivery systems?
- What are the three major classifications of liquid colloidal dispersions, and what distinguishes each from the others?
- What changes in the dispersion medium positively and negatively affect colloidal stability?
- What steps may be taken to avoid destabilizing colloidal dispersions?

Liquid dosage forms: Solutions and disperse systems

Until this point, we have limited discussion to simple solvents, simple solutes (powders), and simple solutions. Recall that solutions are one of several types of liquid dosage forms. Solutions were defined as liquid dosage forms where the solute(s) are dispersed on a molecular level, then were dissolved. Solutions are normally highly stable delivery systems because this molecular dispersion provides a fairly unchanging environment. Stability is also imparted to solutions because they are thermodynamically favorable.

The thermodynamic stability of liquid drug delivery systems is dependent on molecular interactions – the interactions of adhesion and cohesion (refer to the discussion in Chapter 3). Recall that a solute will spontaneously enter a solution if adhesive forces (those between dissimilar components) are greater than cohesive forces (those between similar components). If the attractive forces between the solvent and solute exceed solute–solute and solvent–solvent forces, formation of a solution is favorable. The reverse process (the solution separating into separate solute and solvent phases) is then unfavorable. Since, by definition, solutions have become homogeneous mixtures, the thermodynamic drive for solute to leave the solution is small, unless an environmental parameter, such as temperature, is altered. In Chapter 5 the thermodynamics of liquid drug delivery systems, especially as temperature and surface/interfacial tension relate to them, were discussed.

What is done if a solid is not suitably soluble in a desired (e.g., 'safe') solvent? Or what if a drug were suitably soluble in a liquid medium but the resulting oral dosage form would have an undesirable taste to patients? What if a liquid solute needs to be delivered in a liquid solvent but the two are immiscible? When situations such as these arise, the use of solutions may no longer be a viable option but other liquid dosage forms may be appropriate alternatives. A remedy for these situations often is the use of disperse systems, or simply 'dispersions'.

Components of disperse systems

Disperse systems are composed of two heterogeneous components, the dispersion medium and the dispersed phase, where the two have differing composition, or state. The dispersion medium is also referred to as the external or continuous phase, while the dispersed phase is referred to as the internal or discontinuous phase. The two components can be considered loosely as analogs of the components of solutions – the dispersed phase as the solute and the dispersion medium as the solvent – only dissolution has not occurred in disperse systems.

Solvent ≡ dispersion medium (continuous phase)
Solute ≡ dispersed phase (discontinuous phase)

Key Point

A disperse system contains an external – or continuous – phase and an internal – or discontinuous – phase. The discontinuous phase is the one dispersed in the dispersion medium.

Technically, internal and external phases of dispersions can be composed of gases, liquids or solids. Disperse systems have larger dispersed particle sizes than do solutions. Within disperse systems, coarse dispersions tend to possess larger particle sizes than do colloids. Most pharmaceutical dispersions are solids in liquids or liquids in liquids. Dispersions can be classified based on the dispersed phases' sizes, divided into the two major types, colloidal dispersions, and coarse dispersions. Coarse dispersions are further subdivided into two classifications, suspensions and emulsions. A suspension is composed of a solid dispersed phase in a liquid dispersion medium, whereas an emulsion is composed of a liquid dispersed phase in a liquid dispersion medium (Table 4.1). Coarse dispersions will be discussed further in Chapter 7. Colloidal dispersions have smaller particle sizes than coarse dispersions and are usually composed of solid dispersed phases in a liquid dispersion medium (for pharmaceutical uses). The main emphasis of this chapter is on colloidal dispersions. However, much of the matter presented regarding colloidal dispersions has application to coarse dispersion systems as well.

Liquid colloids are dispersions of 'solute' in 'solvent', only not at a molecular level, and dissolution into the bulk medium does not occur. Thus, these are not colloidal solutions but rather colloidal dispersions.

Colloidal dispersions

Solutions contain solvents and solutes of molecular-level sizes. Another method of visualizing solutions is to say they possess 'particles' under one nm (<1 nm) in diameter. Colloidal dispersions are composed of particles whose diameters range from 10 to 1000 nm (1 μm). These particles are larger than ions and molecules, but not so large that the components of colloidal dispersions necessarily separate due to the influence of gravity, as they normally resist this. Colloidal particles are too small to be visible to the naked eye, though some may be viewed with a microscope. Thus, colloids constitute particle sizes that fall between homogeneous mixtures (solutions) and larger heterogeneous mixtures (suspensions and emulsions). Colloidal particles may consist of many types of atoms, ions or molecules. Some molecules may be relatively large, an example being hemoglobin (approximately 6.5 × 5.5 × 5.0 nm). Some commonly encountered colloids include fog (a liquid dispersed in a gas), smoke (a solid dispersed in a gas), whipped cream (a gas dispersed in a liquid), milk (a liquid dispersed in a liquid), paint (a solid dispersed in a liquid), marshmallows (a gas dispersed in a solid) and butter (a liquid dispersed in a solid). Colloidal dispersions offer an alternative formulation strategy for delivery systems that, for physical reasons, or palatability issues, preclude the use of solutions. A drawback of dispersed systems is their proclivity toward thermodynamic instability. Lyophobic colloids (discussed below) tend to have this attribute.

Thermodynamic instability of some dispersions contributes to the tendency of components to separate, coagulate or settle. The intermolecular interactions between the dispersed phases and their dispersion media cause some disperse systems to teeter precariously near instability. It is important to understand the contributing factors to stability and instability if these delivery systems are to be successfully employed. Therefore, emphasis is placed on the major mechanisms by which each type of colloidal system is stabilized, as well as conditions that can lead to destabilization.

Colloids are divided into three types based on the affinity (or lack of it) between the particles of the dispersed phase and those of the dispersion medium. These are lyophobic, lyophilic and association colloids. The small particle size of colloids means they possess large interfacial areas, so colloids are systems in which interfacial properties play important roles. The presence or absence of intermolecular interactions plays an important role in colloidal stability as well. Because of their small particle size, true colloids, like true solutions, tend to remain dispersed due to Brownian motion.

Key Point

The major concern for colloids is destabilization, which can lead to coagulation.

Therefore, in general, settling of colloids in containers is a minor consideration. It will be seen that this is not the case for suspensions and emulsions, which have larger dispersed phase sizes leading to problems of settling or separation. The most important goal pertaining to colloids is to keep them from coagulating (or aggregating). So, a 'stable' colloid is one that remains properly dispersed. Coagulation of colloids can occur with changes in temperature, pH, or electrolyte concentration in the dispersion medium. Coagulated colloids are virtually impossible to redisperse, once coagulation has occurred. Obviously, for drug delivery systems, coagulation of colloids must be avoided. Beneficial coagulation of colloids is encountered everyday, and includes yogurt, whey, cheeses, and the treatment of wastewater. Drug delivery systems are not normally designed where coagulation is an intended, helpful attribute. So, how are colloids made stable?

Three types of colloids

Lyophobic ('dispersion phase hating') colloids cannot directly rely on stabilizing attributes of their dispersion media. Lyophilic ('dispersion phase loving') colloids do receive stabilization from the dispersion medium. If the colloidal delivery system employs an aqueous-based dispersion medium, the 'lyo' is replaced with 'hydro,' and the two colloidal systems are referred to as hydrophobic and hydrophilic colloids, respectively. Association colloids are composed of collections of amphiphilic molecules and/or ions, and differ significantly from lyophobic and lyophilic colloids. Therefore, association colloids will be discussed in a separate section of this chapter.

What are some colloidal systems with which we deal? These include gels, magmas, sols, and milks. The particle size range is fairly broad for each of these dosage forms, ranging from solution to suspension particle sizes. For this chapter, references made will pertain to those of colloidal size.

A gel is a semisolid system composed of either small inorganic or large organic molecules in a liquid dispersion medium. It is a colloidal system that, under correct conditions of concentration and temperature, 'sets' into a solid or semisolid form. The semisolid formed differs from what is meant by the term 'coagulated' as the semisolid is intentionally created and reversible. The rigidity of a gel is due to an intertwining network of the dispersed phase, which traps the dispersion medium. Gels that contain dispersed phases in the colloidal range are often called magmas or milks. By convention, milks and magmas are aqueous-based and have larger dispersed particle sizes than do other gels.

'Sol' is a general term used primarily for dispersions of solids in liquids, but is also used to refer to dispersions in solid or gaseous media. Hydrosols are dispersions in water, alcosols are dispersion in alcohols and aerosols are dispersions in air or a gas.

Lyophilic colloids are thermodynamically stable systems, possessing extensive interactions between the dispersed phase and the dispersion medium. As stated above, 'lyo' means 'solvent or dispersion medium.' The dispersed phases of lyophilic colloids are composed of single macromolecules. These macromolecules have strong stabilizing interactions with their dispersion media. If the dispersion medium is aqueous, hydrophilic is more descriptive (Figure 6.1).

Once lyophilic colloidal dispersions are formed they are reversible. Lyophilic colloids exhibit attractive (adhesional) forces between the two phases. The attraction between the dispersed particles and the dispersion medium provides a stabilizing effect on the system. So, lyophilic colloids have a lower tendency to coagulate

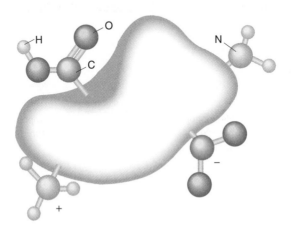

Figure 6.1 Hydrophilic colloid

Hydrophilic groups attached to a colloidal particle can help particle stability by adding more repulsion between particles via electrostatic forces.

than lyophobic colloids. Hydration is the major mechanism for stabilizing hydrophilic colloids. Hydration is the attraction of the dispersed particles to water in the dispersion medium. Since the two phases (dispersed and dispersion phases) do interact attractively in this type of system, water creates a protective sheath around the colloidal particles. This should be differentiated from dissolution. The dispersed phase particles here remain a separate entity. To displace this protective 'water' sheath that surrounds the particles, a large amount of energy is required, so hydrophilic colloids tend to be very stable. Therefore, some attraction between the particles and water, along with repulsion among dispersed particles, provides overall stability to hydrophilic colloids. In other words, the presence of both adhesive and cohesive interactions provides a robust mechanism by which particles of the dispersed phase are maintained in a dispersed state, keeping hydrophilic colloids stable. The favorable thermodynamic properties allow the formation of lyophilic (hydrophilic, if the dispersion medium is aqueous) colloids to be spontaneous. Hydrophilic colloids are stabilized via both hydration of the dispersed particles and electrical repulsion between the particles themselves. When part of a more complex delivery system, hydrophilic colloids exhibit a dramatic increase in the system viscosity with increasing concentration. Examples of hydrophilic colloids that exhibit this behavior are gelatin and methylcellulose.

Lyophobic colloids, in contrast (to lyophilic colloids), are actually stabilized via repulsion between dispersed particles and the dispersion medium (Figure 6.2).

Lyophobic (hydrophobic if an aqueous dispersion medium) colloids are large collections of ions and are thermodynamically unstable systems, possessing little stabilizing interaction between the dispersed phase and the dispersion medium due to low adhesional forces between the two phases. Lyophobic colloids do not form spontaneously, but rather require special techniques to create them. Stability for lyophobic colloids is achieved through ensuring balanced repulsion both within the dispersed phase

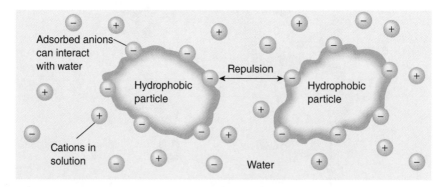

Figure 6.2 Adsorbed ions acting to stabilize hydrophobic colloidal particles

Ions can sometimes be adsorbed onto the dispersed particle surface, providing repulsion (V_R involves mainly electrostatic repulsion forces, discussed later in this chapter) among dispersed particles and imparting a degree of attraction between the hydrophobic dispersed phase and the dispersion medium. Both repulsive and attractive forces are necessary to provide stability to this type of colloid.

and between the dispersed phase and dispersion medium. Hydrophobic colloids are stabilized only through electrical repulsion among particles – and between particles and the aqueous dispersion medium. When part of a more complex delivery system, hydrophobic colloids do not alter the system viscosity with increasing concentration. Examples of hydrophobic colloids are silver iodide and gold sols.

Association (or amphiphilic, meaning solvent and solute 'loving') colloids are thermodynamically stable systems in which the dispersed phase consists of aggregates of amphiphilic molecules or ions (micelles) that have strong interactions between the dispersed phase and dispersion medium, and so can act as surfactants (Figure 6.3). These colloids possess hydrophilic and hydrophobic regions within the same molecule, which allow the favorable interactions with the dispersion medium and the dispersed phase. Aqueous-based association colloids are stabilized via both hydration of the dispersed particles and by hydrophobic interactions that create micelles. At low dispersed phase concentrations, the molecules exist in true solution (Figures 6.4 and 6.5). At higher concentrations, they spontaneously aggregate above the critical micelle concentration (CMC) to form micelles.

When part of a more complex delivery system, hydrophilic colloids exhibit little change in viscosity, though some increase the delivery system viscosity when at high concentrations. Examples of aqueous association colloids are those created with Tween 80 and bile salts.

The common characteristic of all types of colloids is the interaction between the dispersed phase and the dispersion medium. When controlled, any type can remain dispersed. Controlling colloidal dispersions depends on maintaining optimum balances of attractive and repulsive forces between phases. Therefore, we will take a closer look at these forces. Lyophilic and lyophobic colloids will be discussed first, followed by association colloids.

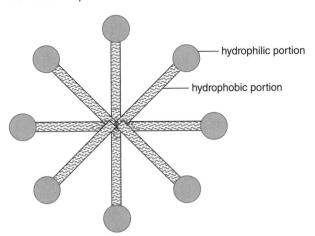

hydrophilic portion

hydrophobic portion

Figure 6.3 Cross-section of a micelle

In this illustration, the long portions are hydrophobic, while the small balls are hydrophilic. When dispersed at lower concentrations (below the critical micelle concentration), these amphiphiles can act as surfactants, stabilizing colloidal dispersions.

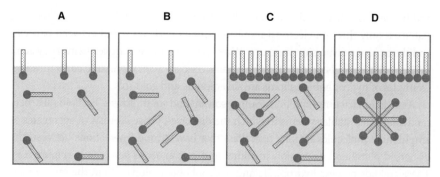

Figure 6.4 Increasing amphiphile concentration creates micelles

In (A), the concentration of amphiphile is below the critical micelle concentration (CMC). As amphiphile concentration increases, (B) illustrates a concentration of amphiphile still below the CMC, and (C) at a point where the dispersion phase surface is saturated. After surface saturation (above the CMC), amphiphiles form micelles in order to minimize potential energy (D).

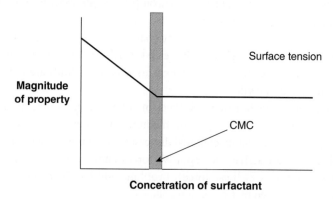

Figure 6.5 Amphiphile (surfactant) concentration and critical micelle concentration (CMC)

As the surfactant concentration increases, surface tension decreases until the CMC is reached. After the CMC is reached, no further decrease in surface tension occurs because the interface is saturated.

Stabilizing forces for colloids

I. Lyophilic and lyophobic colloids

As mentioned, the dispersed phase and dispersion medium of lyophobic colloids do not interact well with regard to stabilizing the system. The result is that not only can these colloids be difficult to make, but they also are sensitive to surrounding conditions, such as changing ionic strength or pH. The stability of any colloidal system requires keeping the dispersed phase dispersed (i.e., not coagulated). Therefore, the dispersed phase should not be overly attracted to either the dispersion medium (adhesion) or the other dispersed particles (cohesion). The condition of being dispersed creates a thermodynamic instability: the dispersed particles possess potential energy (PE) that is not difficult to lose. By aggregating with other particles this PE is lost, but then so is our drug delivery system. Lyophobic colloids have a propensity to coagulate in order to gain thermodynamic stability, and this is not what we wish to occur. In order for disperse drug delivery systems to be successful, they must remain in a dispersed condition. Dispersed particles of hydrophobic colloids (the most common useful type of lyophobic colloids) have a natural lack of affinity for water, and so have a drive to separate from the water. They can be prepared in water only if stabilized in some way – either by adsorption of ions onto their surfaces or by providing hydrophilic groups, that will interact positively with water, to their surfaces. This allows a modicum of affinity for the dispersion medium, offsetting the natural attraction between particles, hopefully adequate to keep the dispersed particles apart. Hydrophobic colloids do not spontaneously disperse in aqueous media (as hydrophilic colloids do). So, providing some measure of affinity for water, as well as ensuring colloidal particles repel each other, provides dispersion and stability.

Disperse systems can be viewed as balances of potential energy. Keep in mind this is applicable to all disperse systems, including colloids, suspensions and emulsions. For now, the discussion is focused on colloids. What are the attractive and repulsive forces at work? Attractive forces include van der Waals interactions and the electrical attractions between disparately charged particles or portions of particles. Repulsive forces include electrical repulsion between particles or portions of particles for any colloid type. Also, steric hindrance is a repulsive force. In some instances, steric effects due to the actions of components intentionally added to the colloidal preparation can add resistance to particle aggregation. For hydrophilic and association colloids, hydration (stabilization via proximal water molecules) of particles and solvation actions (even though a solution is not made) upon particles are contributing forces. A simple mathematical representation of the interacting forces on colloidal particles can be represented using the following general equation:

$$V_T = V_A + V_R + V_S$$

where

V_T = the total (net) force

V_A = the total of attractive forces (van der Waals, adsorbed ions)

V_R = the electrostatic repulsive forces

V_S = steric repulsion.

V_A is traditionally a negative value, indicating attraction. V_R and V_S are traditionally positive values, indicating repulsion.

To illustrate the actions of those forces applicable to hydrophobic colloids, Figures 6.6 to 6.9 are used. The forces result in PEs of attraction and repulsion, along with a net PE along the distance from a charged particle's surface. The net force between particles and dispersion medium, V_T, is the resulting sum of forces that attract the particles to the dispersion medium, attract particles to one another, and those that repel particles from the dispersion medium and those forcing repulsion between particles (Figure 6.6). For a stable dispersion, the goal is to achieve a V_T as close to zero as possible (i.e., no net force). A closer look at the interparticulate (cohesive) forces of the dispersed particles will be taken.

Keeping the dispersed phase particles apart is a major requirement for disperse systems. The distance at which particles are kept is the heart of this requirement. Two charged particles (any dispersion type, but for now colloidal particles) can be viewed as possessing both attractive and repulsive forces between them, as illustrated in Figures 6.7 to 6.9. The steric forces (V_s) act over a fairly definite range

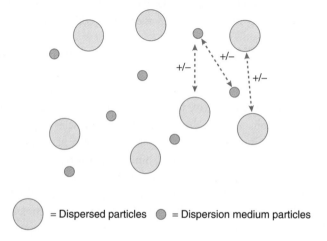

$\bigcirc$ = Dispersed particles $\bullet$ = Dispersion medium particles

Figure 6.6 Attractive and repulsive forces acting in disperse systems

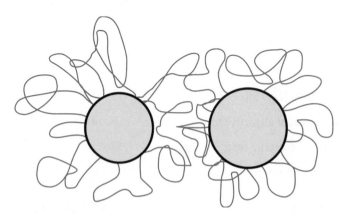

Figure 6.7 Steric forces acting among particles

This is part of V_s = steric repulsive forces. Attaching a lyophobic substance to colloidal particles can physically inhibit close approach of other dispersed phase particles (steric hindrance).

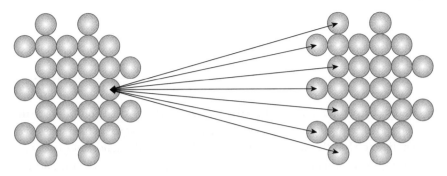

Figure 6.8   van der Waals attractive forces acting among particles

This is part of V_A = the total of van der Waals attractive forces. Note that pair interactions are additive. The additive effect of pair interactions is a reason why (especially) lyophobic colloids tend to coagulate. The result of V_A (van der Waals attraction illustrated) can either be stabilizing or destabilizing, depending on the strength of interactions. If V_A is too strong, coagulation of dispersed particles can result.

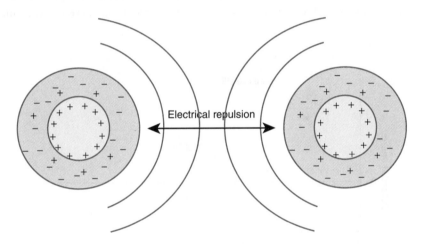

Electrical repulsion

Figure 6.9   Electrostatic repulsive forces between lyophobic colloidal particles

This is part of V_R = electrostatic repulsive forces. Represented here are particles with a surface charge, with ions surrounding each particle, in a 'diffuse area'. If colloidal particles naturally are charged, this can add stability to the particles by preventing coagulation. Obviously, changing the medium pH, or adding electrolytes, can affect V_R. Represented here are positively charged colloidal particles surrounded by a layer of similarly and oppositely charged ions. The 'core' charge of the colloidal particles acts through this 'diffuse layer,' causing particles to repel one another. As will be described, two positively charged particles (colloids for the present discussion) will be most stable at a specific distance from each other. At this distance, particles are attracted by the 'diffuse areas' around their counterparts, while balancing attractions with repulsion between the positive charges of the actual particles.

and remain relatively constant. The electrical forces (V_A, V_R), however, vary in their net action on two charged particles, depending on the distance between the charged particles.

Key Point

> Attractive forces between dispersed particles (V_A) act over greater distances than do repulsive forces (V_R).

The electrical repulsive and attractive forces (V_A and V_R) that contribute to the net force (V_T) acting between two charged particles are unequal in the ranges over which they act. It is this disparity of range that presents the major complexity for disperse systems: what is the 'best' distance to keep particles, and can the particles actually be kept at that distance? Attractive forces act over longer ranges than do repulsive forces: the PE of attractive forces declines with inverse proportion to r^6, whereas repulsive forces decline with inverse proportion to r^9, where r is distance between molecules. The disparate PEs (normally in units of millivolts, mV) are graphed in Figure 6.10, along with the net PE.

By convention, attractive PE is assigned a negative value, while repulsive PE is assigned positive values. By plotting $1/r^9$, a typical repulsion curve representing

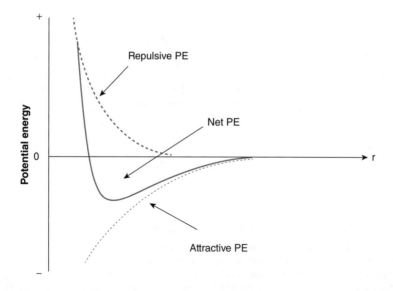

Figure 6.10 Ranges of interparticulate attractive and repulsive forces acting on charged particles

When two like-charged particles are considered, it is found that forces of attraction (V_A) act at distances longer than do repulsive forces (V_R, V_S). The net potential energy (PE; V_T) is repulsive at very close range, while attractive forces dominate at intermediate distances, becoming equal (both declining to zero) at larger ranges. These variations in dominant forces are reflected in the net potential energy. Where the net PE is minimized are distances at which charged particles are most likely to reside, while still remaining, to some degree, separated. These PE minima are also referred to as PE wells, and are distances at which dispersed particles will be most stable. Not shown is a second net PE minimum, further away, which will be discussed later in this chapter.

the PE of repulsion (related to V_R) is created, and is labeled 'repulsive PE.' The plot of $-1/r^6$ represents the attractive PE at varying distances between the two charged particles, representing the attractive PE, V_A. Finally, the plot of difference between the attractive and repulsive functions results in the net PE values, related to V_T.

Key Point

> There are specific distances where net potential minima occur, where particles are most likely to reside, and result in the most stable dispersed systems.

Figure 6.10 is important because it reveals that, as a result of the differing ranges of forces, there is a certain separation distance that offers the most overall electrical stability to charged particles, based on the net PE at these separation distances. This is a PE well where the net PE is most disparately influenced by attractive forces. For disperse systems there are usually two PE minima, as shown in the embellished Figure 6.11. One minimum (the outer) occurs where there is optimal separation distance between two dispersed particles. This distance is beneficial to stability of the disperse system and is the distance that is preferred because, if a disperse system does decompose but the particles can be held at the outer minimum, the disperse system is energetically much easier to redisperse. The second (inner) PE minimum occurs at a distance between particles that may be detrimental. For colloidal particles, the inner minimum represents such a close approach between two particles that interpenetration of (collision between) the particles is likely. Interpenetration or collision means 'aggregation' or 'coagulation' of the colloid is likely. Recovering from this closer, larger magnitude PE well is difficult, or perhaps even impractical, due to the amount of energy that would be required to overcome the PE barrier. What this illustrates is that, if a dispersed phase is not stabilized at the outer distance where the energy minimum occurs, the resulting coagulation may be irreversible and the dosage form ruined.

Because there is often a propensity toward interpenetration between dispersed phase components, especially in systems of lyophobic colloids, care must be exercised when considering altering conditions of the disperse system. Any part of the delivery system that can inhibit electrical attraction between the dispersed phase and the dispersion medium, or the repulsion between dispersed particles of a hydrophobic colloidal (i.e., added electrolytes), can destabilize the colloid. Other potentially disruptive events that can occur include temperature and pH changes. As hydrophobic particles are repelled by water, one stabilizing effect imparted by water is a repulsive force toward the dispersed particles. However, provided enough impetus in the form of added electrolytes, acids, bases or temperature change, the protection of the dispersed phase can be compromised, and coagulation can yet occur. In the end, the stability of

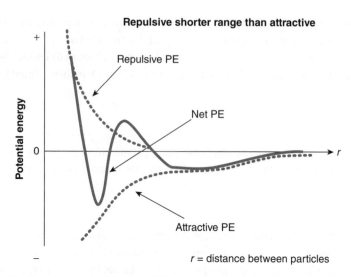

Figure 6.11 Outer net potential energy (PE) well

This figure illustrates that 1) repulsive forces dominate when two charged particles are extremely close – to a point that the energy required to be expended to move the particles closer together makes it very unlikely to occur; 2) the attractive potential is predominant at moderate, but still relatively near distances, with two energy minima; and 3) the net interaction is attraction (at moderate distances). However, if particles get very close (the distance of the inner net energy minimum) there is risk of coagulation, which results from interpenetration of the particles' electrical environments.

colloids – and other disperse systems – is dependent upon keeping the particles of the dispersed phase an optimum distance apart at the second (outermost) net PE minimum, which is visualized in Figure 6.12.

Figure 6.12 illustrates two hydrophobic colloid particles at a stable distance from each other. (Note the stabilizing repulsive surface charges on surfaces of two particles; see Figures 6.9 and 6.12.) In this illustration the particles have positively charged surfaces, and thus conform to the requirement that they not attract one another. Closer inspection reveals a region that contains both positive and negative charges, immediately beyond the particles' charged surfaces, that until now, has been referred to as a 'diffuse area.'

The diffuse region of dispersed particles and the diffuse double layer model

What is this area of both negative and positive ions? First, nomenclature will be assigned. Ions that have the same charge sign as that of the particle surface (in this situation, positive) are called similions. Ions with the opposite charge sign as that of the particle surface (here, negative) are called counterions. The area just beyond the charged particle surface is called the diffuse region. The diffuse region then is composed of both similions and counterions.

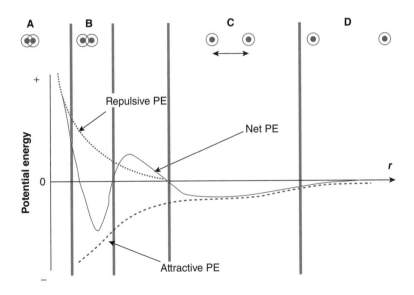

Figure 6.12 Two charged colloidal particles at optimum separation distance

This figure illustrates various proximities of two charged particles in relation to net potential energy (PE). In (A), the particles are so close together they cannot practically be moved any closer. In order for the particles to get this close, a very large amount of energy would need to be applied in order to overcome the large repulsive force. In (B) interpenetration of the diffuse regions of the particles has occurred, meaning for a colloid, aggregation and coagulation. Though this is not desired, it can occur if the interparticulate distance is allowed to fall within the closer PE minimum. In (C), the particles are at an optimum distance for the dosage form, balancing attractive and repulsive PEs and residing in the outer PE minimum. In (D), the particles are too far apart to exert substantial interparticulate interactions.

For disperse systems, the details of how particles sufficiently repel each other are described by the diffuse double layer (DDL) theory and model. The DDL is represented in Figure 6.9 by the more darkly shaded regions surrounding each particle. The DDL contains both counterions and similions.

For the following discussion, the focus is only on one particle and its associated DDL. Also, for the new example a negatively charged particle surface is used. This particle, then, appears as shown in Figure 6.13. Notice an arrow has been placed in the figure, extending from the particle's charged surface through the DDL beyond the particle surface.

The DDL model of the particle above can also be illustrated as if it were overlaid on a graph, as shown in Figure 6.14. In this illustration, the portion of the particle inside the charged surface is represented on the y axis as the dark area on the far left. Since our model particle has associated with it a negative surface charge, this has been represented in contact with the particle, immediately to the left of the y axis. As the charge is associated with the particle, the particle surface is considered to end to the right of the charged surface in the figure. Since there

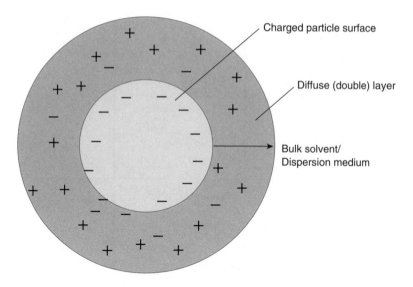

Figure 6.13 The diffuse region and diffuse double layer

Outside a charged particle surface is a region of transition that eventually extends to the bulk solvent/solution. This transition, or double layer contains a gradient of counterions.

is a surface charge associated with the particle, ions near the particle surface will have PE Ψ ('psi', units in mV), with magnitude decreasing with distance along the x axis, away from the particle surface. As ions are either positively or negatively charged, the charged particle surface exerts an attractive or repulsive force acting upon them, respectively. The further away an ion is from the particle surface the lower its PE. In this illustration, negatively charged ions will have a negative (repulsive) potential, whereas positively charged ions will have a positive (attractive) potential. At a certain distance away from the surface of the charged particle, the potentials will fall to zero. Preceding that point, and closer to the particle surface, there is a distance, Ψ_z, which is important with regard to the electrical stability of a colloidal particle, and will be discussed later in this chapter. The entire DDL model is illustrated in Figure 6.14, and will be deconstructed as the discussion proceeds.

In the DDL model, the distinction between the edge of a particle and the beginning of the dispersion medium becomes gradual. The surface charge of the particle is called the 'immobile' phase and is balanced by the equal but opposite charge of the mobile layer of the solvent (this can be viewed as analogous to the diffusion layer described by Fick's Law). The potential (Ψ) developed between the charged particle surface and surrounding ions decreases with distance from the particle surface. The point that is considered the 'end' of the 'diffuse area' is where $\Psi = \Psi_z = \zeta$, the zeta potential. The interactions to be considered also become more numerous.

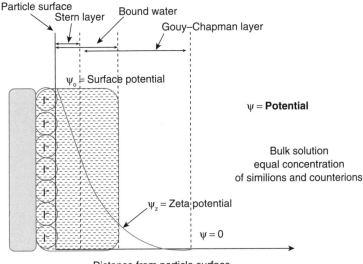

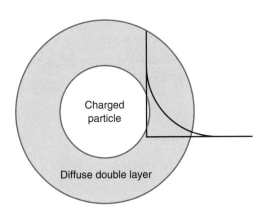

Figure 6.14 The diffuse double layer (DDL) model and plotting potential, Ψ, as a function of distance from the particle surface

The DDL model (top diagram) can be used to describe the relationship between concentration of ions and the distance from the charged particle surface. The lower diagram illustrates, relative to the particle surface, what the plot is representing and where each important point occurs, with respect to the charged particle.

In the present example, adhering to the particle surface are iodide ions (Figure 6.15).

Away from the surface of the particle is a collection of ions generated from sodium iodide and sodium nitrate. The ions include Na^+, I^-, and NO_3^-. In this illustration, Na^+ is a counterion, while I^- and NO_3^- are similions. Overall, the colloidal dispersion must be electrically neutral, but locally, such as in the DDL, regions may be electrically charged. The DDL is the region surrounding the particle that

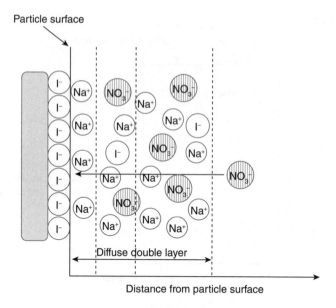

Figure 6.15 The potential (Ψ) of ions in relation to distance from a charged particle surface. Ψ is inversely related to distance from the particle surface.

balances the particle's surface charge. The DDL is itself overall charged as its function is to neutralize the surface charge of the particle (Figure 6.16).

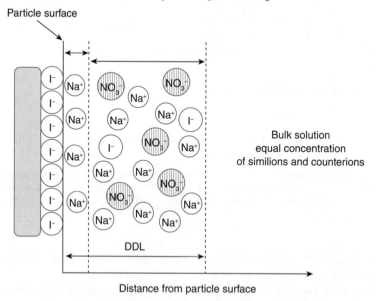

Figure 6.16 Particle surface and the diffuse double layer (DDL)

The DDL (or diffuse double layer) differs from the electrical double layer: the DDL is that portion of the electrical double layer that contains mobile ions (i.e., those not associated with the charged particle surface).

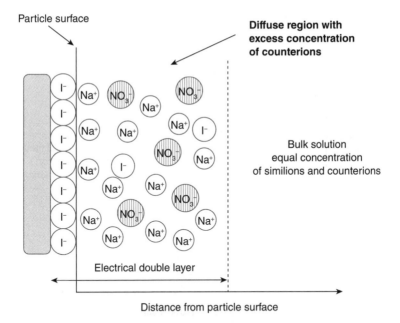

Figure 6.17   The diffuse region and electrical double layer

The diffuse region is synonymous with the diffuse double layer, containing the mobile similions and counterions that ultimately counterbalance the surface charge of the particle.

Beyond the DDL is the bulk solution, which is overall electrically neutral as the system as a whole cannot be electrically charged (positively or negatively). The region between the particle surface and the bulk solution is also known as the diffuse region (Figure 6.17), which contains more counterions than similions in order to provide the necessary overall charge balance. Together, the charged particle surface and diffuse region are called the electrical double layer (not to be confused with the DDL). Therefore, the DDL includes the electrical double layer. The DDL, also called the diffuse layer, is so named because of the mobility of ions within the region. The electrical double layer (Figure 6.17) includes the regions from the particle surface all the way out into the bulk dispersion medium, and has an overall neutral charge. Next, we look more closely at the components of the DDL.

Components of the diffuse double layer

Within the DDL, closest to the particle surface, there is a region that contains an excess of counterions (Na^+), and is called the Stern layer (Figure 6.18). In the Stern layer, predominantly counterions are held closely to the particle surface.

As mentioned previously, the DDL neutralizes the particle's surface charge, and so is not itself electrically neutral. The DDL's overall charge is opposite to, but balances, the surface charge. Also, as previously mentioned, there is a distance-dependent PE (Ψ)

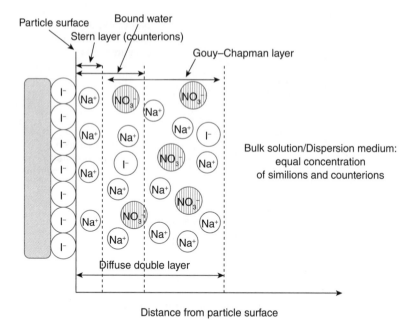

Figure 6.18 The different regions of the diffuse double layer

between similions or counterions and the charged particle surface. Similions have negative (repulsive) PEs, while counterions have positive (attractive) PEs. The next 'layer' further away from the particle surface, beyond the Stern layer is the bound water region (Figure 6.18). Here, the solvent (dispersion medium) is present, along with a mixture of similions and counterions, but the ions in this area are less mobile than in the bulk medium. When ions move in the bound water region, the dispersion medium (water in this example) moves with them.

The edge of the bound water region furthest from the particle is known as the shear plane. The shear plane is the boundary between the environment that will migrate through the dispersion medium with the charged particle, and the environment that will not, and can be revealed by subjecting the disperse system to electrophoresis. The potential at the shear plane is the zeta potential. A sufficiently high zeta potential (meaning, distance away from the colloidal particle surface) ensures a stable disperse system as a result of sufficient repulsion between adjacent particles. Smaller zeta potentials indicate potential instability due to the proximity particles may approach each other.

The portion of the DDL furthest from the particle surface is the Gouy–Chapman layer (Figure 6.14). Since the Stern layer is composed almost exclusively of counterions, most of the particle's surface charge is neutralized by the far end of that layer. The Gouy–Chapman layer contains the bound water region and is a more diffuse region than the Stern layer, containing a greater mix of counterions and similions.

Ionic potential energy and zeta potential

Here, the discussion returns to the importance of the PEs of the similions and counterions, and their relation to the zeta potential. As stated above, negative or positive PE decreases with increasing distance from the charged surface. The PEs also depend on the charge magnitudes of the similions and counterions. If plotted as an overlaid graph (Figure 6.14), this decrease in potential (Ψ) with increasing distance from the particle surface can be seen. Ψ_0 is the potential at the charged surface ($x = 0$), and is the maximum value for potential. Ψ then decays at points further from the charged surface until it reaches a value of zero at the bulk solution (the end of the Gouy–Chapman layer, which is also the end of the DDL). There is a large Ψ decrease in the Stern layer where there is an abundance of counterions.

We return to Figure 6.14 to illustrate the meaning of the important value of zeta potential – now understood to be Ψ_ζ. Zeta potential is an important parameter for determining the thickness of the mobile components of a colloidal particle, and therefore the particle's stability – or tendency toward coagulation – can be assessed. The simplified plot is illustrated in Figure 6.18, although the plot shown in Figure 6.19 is easier to read, understand and apply.

The potential (Ψ) at varying distances from the particle surface is not readily measurable. However, the zeta potential (ζ, shear plane) can be indirectly

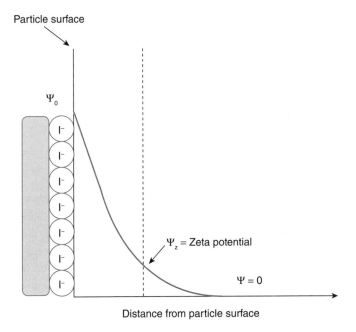

Figure 6.19 Illustration of zeta potential in relation to a charged particle surface

The zeta potential is a useful parameter to help predict the mobile layer thickness, and therefore the potential stability of colloidal particles.

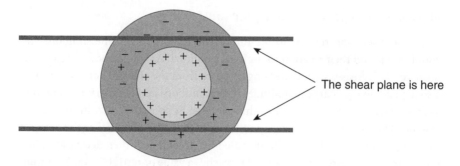

Figure 6.20 Shear plane and zeta potential

If placed in an electrophoretic field, charged colloidal particles will migrate, bringing with them a portion of the diffuse double layer (to the shear plane). Since zeta potential is also a measurement of the mobile layer thickness, both the shear plane (electrophoresis) and zeta potential are informative/predicative of colloidal particle stability.

quantified using electrophoresis, where particle migration rate is a function of the zeta potential. Figure 6.20 illustrates what is occurring with a hypothetical charged colloidal particle in an electrophoretic environment. The particle moves in an electrophoretic field, bringing with it some, but not all, of the diffuse region. The shear plane (the area from the particle surface through the bound water layer) is the defining line between the portion of the particle and DDL that moves and the portion that does not move in the electric field. Thus, the shear plane physically is the zeta potential, and is measured in mV.

Key Point

The zeta potential links electrical potential with shear plane thickness (mV ≈ Å).

Usefulness of zeta potential

What do these measurements tell us? What is a 'stable' predictive value? Since millivolts of potential can be equated to mobile layer thickness, there can be an accepted minimum above which a colloid can be considered stable. Disperse systems with zeta potentials greater than about +/−25 mV are typically stable systems. The DDL and zeta potential are related in that reduction or enlargement of one implies a similar change in the other. Why are the zeta potential and DDL thickness important considerations with regard to dispersed systems? If a constituent is added to the disperse system that reduces the zeta potential (decreases the thickness of the DDL), there is a correspondingly increased risk of coagulation or precipitation of the dispersed phase. In this chapter, the focus is on colloidal dispersions, but the causes of degradations of all disperse systems follow the same,

Coagulation

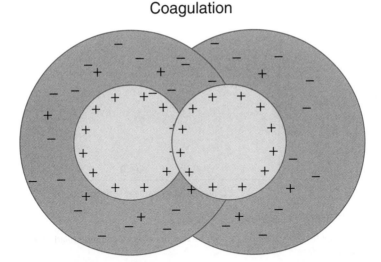

Figure 6.21 Coagulation of colloidal particles

This figure illustrates what we are trying to avoid: interpenetration of particles to the point of coagulation. If the protective sheath surrounding a charged particle surface is compromised, the result can be interpenetration of diffuse regions, and coagulation of the system.

or similar, rules. A decrease in zeta potential values indicates there is less protection accorded the dispersed phase by the protective sheath of the DDL. This allows other particles of the dispersed phase to approach at proximities that allow for interpenetration of the DDLs, enabling the attractive forces to overwhelm the repulsive forces between particles, and result in irreversible coagulation of the (colloidal) particles (Figure 6.21). A sufficiently high zeta potential ensures a stable dispersed system by causing repulsion of adjacent particles. The questions then become: 1) 'How thick is the DDL (what is the Ψ_ζ)?'; 2) 'What can be done to protect Ψ_ζ?'; and 3) 'How can the effects of added electrolytes be predicted?'

Thickness of the diffuse double layer

It has been established that a major objective for maintaining a stable (colloidal) system is to preserve the thickness of the DDL. In other words, we wish to avoid adding anything to the system, such as ions, that would cause the DDL/Ψ_ζ to diminish. The question may arise as to how thick the DDL is. Calculation of the size of the DDL is illustrated in Figure 6.22.

The thickness of the DDL is an important parameter to know as it directly relates to the stability of the colloidal system. The Ψ plot has been presented previously, but now the equation relating distance from the particle surface to Ψ (which is simply a first-order decay equation) will be considered. The DDL thickness can be calculated using the equation for the plot:

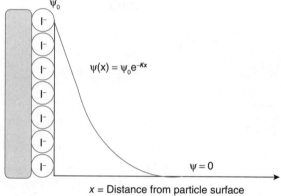

Figure 6.22 Potential (Ψ) as a function of distance

The curve representing the potential (Ψ) can be described by an equation relating Ψ to distance from the particle surface.

$$\Psi_x = \Psi_0 e^{-Kx}$$

where

      x is the distance from the particle surface, in angstroms (Å)
      Ψ_0 is the potential at the particle surface
      K is the Debye constant, with units of Å^{-1} ($1/K$ is the Debye–Hückel length (or simply the Debye length) in Å).

When $x = 1/K$, Ψ has fallen to 37% of Ψ_0 (because when $x = 1/K$, $e^{-(K)(1/K)} = e^{-1}$ $= 0.367$ or 36.7%) and $\Psi_x = \Psi_0 e^{-1} = \Psi_0 (0.367) = 1/K$, the Debye length. Often Ψ_ζ is the same as $1/K$, but this is not always true. It has been found that the thickness of the double layer is usually approximately 1.5 K^{-1} (Figure 6.23).

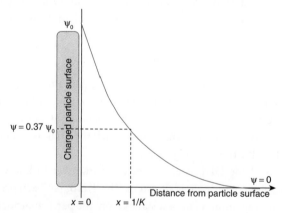

Figure 6.23 Calculation of Debye–Hückel length

The Debye–Hückel length ($1/K$) can be estimated as 37% of Ψ_0.

Key Point

The Debye length, $1/K$, is normally 10–1000 Å for colloidal particles.

$1/K$ ranges from 10–1000 Å; note this size range is in agreement with what was stated as the size of most colloidal particles. What affects the value '$1/K$'?

Clearly, maintaining the Debye length ($1/K$) is key to keeping a dispersed system from degrading. Allowing this distance to shrink will jeopardize the stability of the system by increasing the likelihood particles will interpenetrate, move to the primary PE well, and coalesce or coagulate. How can we predict if this may be a problem with a dispersed system? One approach is to calculate what the 'critical' concentration of added electrolyte will be. This calculation provides a theoretical concentration, and other factors may come into play. There are many methods – all mathematically related – of expressing K and $1/K$. $1/K$ can be expressed as the relationship shown in the equation below. Qualitatively, it can be seen that adding electrolytes to the system risks decreasing the size of the DDL. Furthermore, the valence of the ions added has its effect squared. It can also be observed that temperature plays an important role in colloidal stability: increasing the temperature of the colloid also decreases the DDL thickness. These parameters are represented by the following equation:

$$\frac{1}{K}(cm) = \sqrt{\frac{\varepsilon\varepsilon_0 kT}{2CN_A z^2 e^2}}$$

For the dimensional analysis, the value of $1/K$ using the above equation is in centimeters (cm):

$$\frac{1}{K} = \sqrt{\frac{\left(\dfrac{C^2}{N.m^2}\right)\left(\dfrac{m}{100\,cm}\right)\left(\dfrac{N.m}{J}\right)\left(\dfrac{J}{K}\right)K}{\left(\dfrac{moles}{L}\right)\left(\dfrac{1}{mole}\right)\left(\dfrac{L}{1000\,cm^3}\right)\left(charge^2\right)\left(\dfrac{C}{charge}\right)^2}} = \sqrt{cm^2} = cm$$

where

$1/K =$ the Debye–Hückel (or simply, 'Debye') length

$\varepsilon_0 =$ electric permittivity in a vacuum $= \dfrac{8.85419 \times 10^{-12}\, C^2}{N.m^2}$ (C = coulombs, N = newtons, m = meters)

$\varepsilon =$ dielectric constant of the solvent (dispersion medium) – dimensionless

$k =$ Boltzmann constant $= 1.38 \times 10^{-23}$ m²/kg²K (m² per kg² × kelvin)

$\quad = \dfrac{1.38065 \times 10^{-23}\, J}{K}$ (J = joules, K = kelvin)

T = temperature, K (kelvin)

C = concentration of a given ion/electrolyte (mol/L)

N_A = Avogadro's number (6.022×10^{-23}/mole)

z = valence of a given ion (charge) (counterion)

e = charge of an electron = 1.0622×10^{-19} C (coulombs).

This equation provides Debye lengths in cm, which can be converted to Å, if desired. To provide correct units, the following conversions should be added to the equation:

$$\frac{1}{K} = \sqrt{\frac{\varepsilon\varepsilon_0 \left(\dfrac{m}{100\,cm}\right)\left(\dfrac{N.m}{J}\right)kT}{2CN_A \left(\dfrac{1L}{1000\,cm^3}\right)z^2 e^2}}$$

A factor (10^8 Å/cm) can be added so that $1/K$ will be in Å:

$$\frac{1}{K}(\text{Å}) = \sqrt{\frac{\varepsilon\varepsilon_0 kT (10^{16})}{2CN_A z^2 e^2}} \quad \text{or} \quad \frac{1}{K}(\text{Å}) = (10^{16}) \times \sqrt{\frac{\varepsilon\varepsilon_0 kT}{2CN_A z^2 e^2}} = \text{Å}$$

For $z = 1$, the calculated Debye lengths for specified electrolyte concentrations are shown in the Table 6.1. Note how, by increasing electrolyte concentration, the Debye length – and therefore the double layer thickness – decreases. This illustrates how increasing counterion concentration of a disperse system can lead to unstable Debye lengths (DDL thickness) and coagulation. In this example, an increase of the $z = 1$ counterion concentration from 0.00001 M to 0.001 M compromises the DDL by 90%.

If a similar relationships were illustrated when $z > 1$ the effects of the square of the counterion valence would be even more evident.

As might be anticipated then, the addition of electrolytes (salts, acids or bases) to a colloid can reduce $1/K$ and eventually causes aggregation or flocculation. Even addition of a 1:1 electrolyte to a colloidal system can cause profound changes in the Debye length. Since the effect is related to the square of the valence, multivalent

Table 6.1 Selected calculated Debye lengths	
Molar concentration of $z = 1$ electrolyte	Resulting calculated Debye length (cm and Å)
10^{-7} M	10^{-4} cm (10,000 Å)
10^{-5} M	10^{-5} cm (1000 Å)
10^{-3} M	10^{-6} cm (100 Å)

counterions can easily be devastating to disperse system stability. Stabilizing agents are sometimes added to colloids in order to prevent aggregation. Stabilizing agents can act via steric effects (Figure 6.7), but also through effects on the zeta potential.

Counterions in practice

What about practical applications though? It is not convenient to measure the Debye thickness. What is more practical is predicting the concentration of counterions that may present problems with stability. The critical concentration, C, can be derived from the calculations above if the minimum stable Debye length of the existing system is known:

$$C = \frac{K^2 \varepsilon \varepsilon_0 kT}{2N_A z^2 e^2}$$

C is the concentration of counterion above which the Debye length reduction would likely destabilize a colloidal dispersion. However, this information may not be easily accessible or measurable. But, even a subjective inspection of the variables of the Debye length equation (as shown above) can illustrate parameters for which one should be wary. Those that are within our control have been mentioned throughout this section, and include temperature, electrolyte concentration and valence of electrolytes.

Lyophobic and lyophilic colloids depend greatly on the balances struck between the dispersed phases and the dispersion media. That lyophilic colloids exhibit favorable interactions (attraction) between the dispersed phases and dispersion media generally results in more stable preparations than do lyophobic colloids. However, both can be used for drug delivery systems, and both require forethought with regard to electrical changes that will possibly impact these preparations.

II. Amphiphilic (association) colloids

As previously discussed, association colloids are composed of aggregates of amphiphilic molecules called micelles. Amphiphilic ('both loving') molecules, many of which are surfactants or surface active agents, possess regions both of hydrophobic and hydrophilic character, imparting acceptable solubility in both environments (Figure 6.24). To be a surfactant, an amphiphile must not be overly soluble in either environment, but must possess some degree of moderation in solubility. Amphiphiles then favorably interact with both hydrophilic and hydrophobic environments simultaneously. To use the terms introduced in Chapter 1, an amphiphilic molecule can possess both polar and nonpolar regions within the one molecule. A common method of illustrating this is to employ the 'ball and stick' diagram (Figure 6.24). The 'ball' represents the polar region of this molecule, while the 'stick' represents the nonpolar region. Though soluble in both

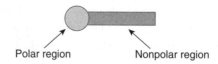

Polar region   Nonpolar region

Figure 6.24   A generic amphiphilic molecule

This is a conceptual illustration of an amphiphile – a molecule possessing some degree of both hydrophilicity and hydrophobicity. More complex amphiphiles can have multiple hydrophilic and hydrophobic regions.

environments, the degree of solubility in each environment is determined by the relative proportion of each type of region. This degree is specific to each amphiphile, and is roughly quantified with the hydrophilic lipophilic balance, or HLB, which is discussed in Chapters 5 and 7. The generic amphiphilic molecule can be altered to emphasize the relative degree of solubility in each environment.

If the illustrated molecule were added to an aqueous environment in low concentration, it would simply rise to the surface of the aqueous environment, orienting its polar regions toward the aqueous environment, with its nonpolar regions exposed at the interface (Figure 6.4). (Note that if a hydrophobic solvent were used, the opposite orientation would occur.) If a hydrophobic liquid were present, the amphiphile would orient so that it would be present in both hydrophilic and hydrophobic environments. This will be especially important for emulsions, which will be discussed in the Chapter 7.

After a sufficient concentration of the amphiphile is added to the medium, the interface will become saturated (Figure 6.4). Beyond this saturation concentration, further addition of the amphiphile will cause the amphiphile to begin orienting in the most energetically favorable way – within the aqueous environment. This aggregation (a positive meaning in this context) of amphiphilic molecules occurs spontaneously and rapidly above its surface saturation concentration, forming micelles. The CMC is the amphiphile concentration where this occurs (Figure 6.4). Micelles become the dispersed phase of an association colloid and are the approximate size to be in the colloidal range. Association colloids only exist when micelles form above the CMC of the amphiphile(s). Of interest regarding micelles is the potential for encasing materials (i.e., drugs) and creating a liquid delivery system in which the dispersed phase is not like the dispersion medium. For example, Figures 6.25 and 6.26 illustrate placing a nonpolar 'solute' in an aqueous environment.

In the system depicted in Figures 6.25 and 6.26, nonpolar solutes (e.g., drugs) can be 'solubilized' by causing them to be entrapped within the hydrophobic region of the amphiphile, within a hydrophilic dispersion medium. (Keep in mind the reverse situation is also possible: entrapment of hydrophilic solutes (drugs) in a hydrophobic amphiphile, within a hydrophobic dispersion medium.) Above the CMC, solutes (drugs) can be entrapped and used in a dispersion medium

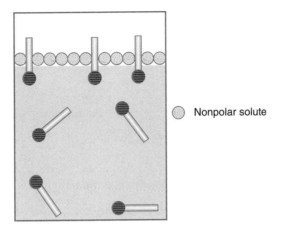

Figure 6.25   Use of colloidal-sized micelles for encasing of nonpolar solutes

The concentration of amphiphile is below the critical micelle concentration, so nonpolar solutes in an aqueous dispersion medium will orient at the dispersion medium's surface (they will float).

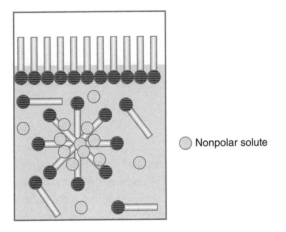

Figure 6.26   Micellar solubilization of a nonpolar solute in association colloid particles

Above the critical micelle concentration, micelles can encapsulate otherwise insoluble materials. Here, the interior of the micelle represents a nonpolar environment. Thus, association colloids can be utilized to act as a 'pseudo-solution,' allowing materials that would otherwise separate to be mixed. In this illustration, colloidal-sized micelles are formed.

dissimilar to the solute (drug). Reasons this may be necessary include physico-chemical considerations for the drug, and to provide improved palatability for oral drug delivery. A graphic representation of this application is shown in Figure 6.27. This figure adds embellishment to Figure 6.5 by adding the presence of an insoluble component to the system.

As would be expected, a lipophilic solute would have very low concentration in a hydrophilic solvent. However, if an amphiphilic component is added, beginning

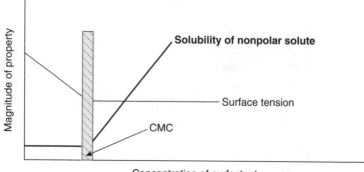

Figure 6.27 Titration of an amphiphile, creating a drug-carrying association colloid

In this illustration an aqueous dispersion medium with a nonpolar dispersed phase is used. As the surfactant (amphiphile) concentration is increased it will eventually reach its critical micelle concentration (CMC), above which colloidal-sized particles are created and dispersed within the aqueous dispersion medium. Nonpolar components can be intentionally entrapped within the micelles. This is often represented by the increased 'solubility' of the nonpolar component ('solubility' meaning 'concentration within the system').

at the amphiphile's CMC, the apparent solubility of the lipophilic solute dramatically increases because an association colloid has been created.

Summary

As colloidal particles are dispersed in the continuous phase, they exhibit Brownian motion. This means they are affected by collisions with molecules of the dispersion medium and tend not to settle. This also imbues colloidal particles with diffusion and colligative properties. Their tendency to diffuse depends on a concentration gradient, and so follows Fick's first law (see Chapter 4).

So, what are the ramifications of all this for a pharmacist? In most instances it is the consideration of what we might want to add (or not add) to an existing dispersed system that causes us (or should cause us) hesitation. With respect to the DDL, addition of ionized substances (counterions) should be of primary concern. As discussed above, careless addition of charged or otherwise ionized substances can alter the zeta potential, leading to unbalancing the sometimes delicate attractive and repulsive forces (intermolecular interactions) between dispersed phase components and/or between dispersed phase and dispersion medium components. The result may be coagulation, coalescence, precipitation, or creaming of the delivery system. Any of these conditions present a high probability the original dispersed system may be irretrievable. Attention should be paid to the potential effects pH changes can have on colloidal particle stability.

Added electrolytes and changes in temperature (especially increases) are the main parameters over which the pharmacist can exert some control. Heat increases the molecular motion of particles, increasing the collision frequency among particles, promoting aggregation. Whenever they adhere following a collision, colloidal particles increase in size until eventually the larger particles settle out of dispersion medium. Added electrolytes (counterions) cause neutralization of surface-adsorbed ions on hydrophobic colloids, and both neutralize surface ions and compete for water of hydration in hydrophilic colloids. These actions also lead to dispersed phase condensation. So, due to temperature and/or electrolyte changes, at some point as indicted before, once the colloid aggregates and settles, it is usually impossible to redisperse.

Self-assessment questions

1. What is a dispersion?

2. What are colloids, or colloidal dispersions, and how do they differ from other liquid drug delivery systems?

3. What is the approximate size of colloidal particles, and how does this differ from particle sizes of other liquid delivery systems?

4. What characteristics make colloidal dispersions unique from other liquid delivery systems?

5. What are the three major classifications of colloidal dispersions, and what distinguishes each from the others?

6. Using the equation for the extent of the DDL $(1/K)$:

$$\frac{1}{K}(cm) = \sqrt{\frac{\varepsilon\varepsilon_0 KT}{2CN_A z^2 e^2}}$$

   What effect does increasing electrolyte concentration have on a colloid?

7. Using the equation for the extent of the DDL $(1/K$, as above) what effect does increasing counterion valence have on a colloid?

8. Using the equation for the extent of the DDL $(1/K$, as above) what do you think is the effect of decreasing dielectric constant on a colloid?

9. Using the equation for the extent of the DDL $(1/K$, as above) what effect does increasing temperature have on a colloid?

10. What steps may be taken to avoid destabilizing colloidal dispersions?

7

Disperse systems – Coarse dispersions – Suspensions and emulsions

Learning objectives

Upon completion of this chapter, you should be able to answer the following questions:

- What is a coarse dispersion?
- What are suspensions, and how do they differ from other liquid drug delivery systems?
- What are emulsions, and how do they differ from other liquid drug delivery systems?
- What is the approximate size of suspension and emulsion dispersed phase particles, and how does this differ from particle sizes of other liquid delivery systems?
- What changes in the dispersion medium positively and negatively affect coarse dispersion stability?
- What steps may be taken to avoid destabilizing coarse dispersions?

In this chapter, the discussion of disperse systems will continue. The focus of Chapter 6 was colloidal dispersions, which are the smallest particle size of dispersed phase within 'disperse systems.' Again, referring to Table 4.1 in Chapter 4, the particle size of the dispersed phase increases from those of solutions, where the 'particle' is in fact dissolved – dispersed at a molecular level ('particle' diameters less than 1.0 nm) – to disperse systems, which have larger particle sizes. Disperse systems are divided into two categories: colloidal dispersions and coarse dispersions. Colloidal dispersions contain the smallest particles that are dispersed, but not truly dissolved (1.0–1000 nm diameter). This imbues colloidal dispersions with some characteristics of both solutions and dispersions, which were described in Chapter 6. Coarse dispersions contain the largest dispersed phase particle sizes (100–50 000 nm diameter) and are further divided into two types: suspensions, in which the dispersed phase is solid, and emulsions, in which the dispersed phase is liquid.

Coarse dispersions

What are the distinguishing characteristics of coarse dispersions? Like fine dispersions, the dispersed phase of coarse dispersions is not necessarily a solid. The dispersion medium and dispersed phase can each be any of the three phases (solid, liquid or gas), though the focus of this text is biased toward those systems that are most commonly used for drug delivery. Water (or aqueous-based liquids) is the most common liquid used for drug delivery systems. As for previous drug delivery systems discussed, water will be the implicit dispersion medium for coarse dispersions. Though the dispersed phase particles of coarse dispersions are larger than those of colloids, many of the same principles apply to both – namely those relying on intermolecular interactions, such as van der Waals' attractive forces and charge- and steric-related repulsive forces. Since coarse dispersions possess larger particles than do solutions and colloidal dispersions, they tend to have greater tendency toward settling and/or separating over time: particles tend to settle to the bottom of a coarse dispersion and liquids (such as oils) tend to rise to the top. In both instances this can mean a delivery system will be rendered useless. Coarse dispersion systems have inherent thermodynamic instability and are constant threats for degradation. But there are methods for preventing and salvaging some coarse dispersions that have gone awry. Therefore, both the variables related to reducing the degradation tendencies of coarse dispersions, and recovering preparations, will be emphasized in this chapter. This chapter is divided into two parts: suspensions and emulsions.

A. Suspensions

What is a 'suspension?' A suspension is a dispersion of solid particles (100–50 000 nm) that are larger than those of colloidal dispersions, but share the trait of insolubility in their dispersion media, which usually is a liquid. Figure 7.1 is a diagram representing a suspension.

Dispersed particles in suspensions are not thermodynamically stable, are acted upon by gravity, and so tend both to adhere to one another and to settle to the bottom of the container. This phenomenon is often unavoidable and can be problematic. For many suspensions it is not a question of if the dispersed phase will settle,

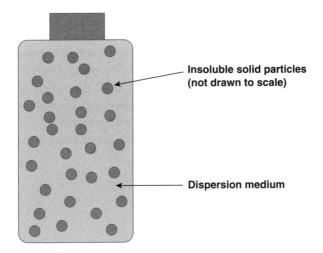

Figure 7.1   Illustration of a suspension

Typically, suspensions are coarse dispersions consisting of solid particles (100–50 000 nm in diameter) in liquid dispersion media.

but rather how quickly and how 'thoroughly' it will settle. The term 'thoroughly' is used here to describe the strength of the interactions among dispersed phase particles when settled. The reader is referred to the discussion of two potential energy (PE) wells in Chapter 6. The concept of PE wells applies to suspensions and emulsions, as well as colloids. The application of this concept is in planning for the inevitability of thermodynamically dictated degradation, but also for models that incorporate alternative forms of disperse systems that allow for degradation to be more readily reversed. Therefore, the main goals for creating the most stable suspensions include: 1) controlling the rate of sedimentation and 2) preventing the development of strong interactions between particles that do sediment. If especially the latter is accomplished, redispersion of the sediment through agitation (shaking the container) is more likely achievable.

Particles and potential energy

To briefly review, when two dispersed particles approach each other, because of inequity between attractive and repulsive forces over distance, there are two net PE 'wells,' or minima, where particles have PE optima (the most energetically stable distances from neighboring particles). The minimum furthest from the neighboring particle requires less energy to leave than does the more proximal minimum. With regard to drug delivery systems, this means particles located at the furthest energy minimum are more easily redispersed than are particles at the closer minimum where they are bound more tightly together.

Particle sedimentation and Stokes' law

As previously mentioned, when particles separate from their dispersion medium, sedimentation of the particles normally occurs. This is not always true, but is the most common scenario. Frequently, then, how quickly the particles settle becomes the variable we wish to control. If settling is slow, measurement and use of the drug delivery system is easier than if particles sediment quickly.

Sedimentation rate of suspension dispersed phases roughly follows Stokes' law:

$$v = \frac{2r^2 \left(\rho_S - \rho_L \right) g}{9 \eta}$$

where

v = sedimentation velocity $(\mathrm{cm \cdot s^{-1}})$
r = particle radius (cm)
ρ_S = density of solid $(\mathrm{g \cdot cm^{-3}})$
ρ_L = density of liquid $(\mathrm{g \cdot cm^{-3}})$
g = gravitational constant $(980.7 \ \mathrm{cm \cdot s^{-2}})$
η = viscosity of the dispersion medium $(\mathrm{poise} = \mathrm{g \cdot cm^{-1} \cdot s^{-1}})$.

Stokes' law operates under the assumption that the particles are small, perfect spheres that create no turbulence and have no collisions (ideal conditions). Within these assumptions, Stokes' law applies to suspensoid concentrations of up to about 2%, and so includes most ophthalmic and injectable suspensions. (Keep in mind that the sedimentation velocity, v, can conceivably be a positive or negative value.) A positive sedimentation velocity indicates a downward particle motion. A negative sedimentation velocity indicates an upward motion. When applying Stokes' law to suspensions the downward (positive) value of v is more often applicable. The discussion of emulsions – the other coarse dispersion – will include application of negative sedimentation velocities, which indicate the dispersed phase is rising. This is a major issue for emulsions, as will be expounded upon later.

Inspection of Stokes' law indicates the suspensoid will settle if its density is greater than that of the dispersion medium, as illustrated in Figures 7.2 and 7.3. If a dispersion medium of greater density than that of the suspensoid were employed, separation by rising to the top of the preparation would be the hazard. If the suspensoid settles in a compact way, a dense cake, which can be difficult to redisperse, may be formed. It is here that the PE well in which the dispersed phase occupies can dictate redispersability. The 'compact' settling of suspensoid demonstrates occupation of the second (closer) PE minimum. This problem will be revisited shortly. For now, it should be kept in mind two issues are important:

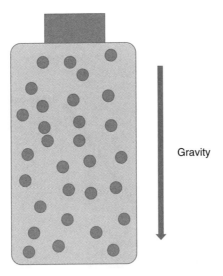

Figure 7.2 Gravity influences suspension particles

The effects of gravity can cause suspensoid particles to settle, the rate of which is described by Stokes' law. The value for sedimentation, v, will be negative, reflecting a downward motion of the dispersed phase. A smaller magnitude of v indicates there will be more time for use of the suspended system before sedimentation occurs.

1) how quickly particles separate, and 2) how strong the interactions among separated particles are.

Key Point

> With regard to suspensions, it important to be mindful of 1) particle sedimentation rates, and 2) strength of sedimented particle interactions (cohesion).

A qualitative examination of Stokes' law reveals a few parameters that can potentially be manipulated to control sedimentation velocity: dispersed particle radius, viscosity of the dispersion medium and possibly the density of the dispersion medium. If the suspended particle size can be reduced (i.e., by trituration), r is reduced, decreasing sedimentation velocity. The viscosity disparity between the dispersion medium and dispersed phase densities may be reduced if the dispersion medium viscosity can be altered or the medium completely changed. This is feasible with regard to preparing drug delivery systems as a whole. Again, this can be done if it does not compromise the safety, efficacy and general physical parameters required by the drug delivery system.

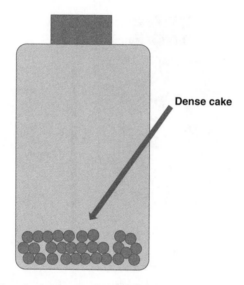

Dense cake

Figure 7.3 Formation of a dense cake due to suspensoid settling

As suspensoid particles settle, they threaten to form a dense cake if particles pack too tightly. This outcome can be avoided if particles are induced to approach each other no closer than the distance represented by the outer energy minimum.

A common solution is to increase the dispersion medium viscosity, decreasing v. One method to increase viscosity is to employ hydrophilic colloids as parts of the coarse dispersions, which have viscosity-increasing properties, as described in Chapter 6. Sometimes apparent solutions to remedy large sedimentation velocities are not helpful though. For example, reduction in suspensoid particle size (if this is a potential option) also increases total dispersed phase surface area, causing Gibbs' free energy (ΔG) to increase:

$$\Delta G = \gamma \Delta A$$

where

   ΔG = free energy change
   γ = interfacial free energy
   ΔA = change in interfacial area.

As the particle size is reduced (such as is accomplished through trituration), the free energy increases. A large free energy indicates that the system is thermodynamically unstable and that it will tend to spontaneously move in the direction of interfacial area reduction (e.g., through crystal growth and/or precipitation) to decrease free energy. Interfacial tension (γ) can be reduced to attempt to offset the increase in surface area, such as by addition of surfactants, but it is unlikely to achieve a large enough impact – one that would completely negate the change in surface area – providing a γ value near 'zero.' Therefore, reducing particle size in an effort to decrease sedimentation rate may sometimes not be helpful. This can also be true for attempts to favorably alter other Stokes' law parameters. It may be impractical to change the density of either the drug (ρ_S) or dispersion medium (ρ_L), so this potential remedy is not commonly employed.

The prior discussion helps understanding that, in many cases, sedimentation of the dispersed phase is going to happen, but it does not mean all is lost. The task is to decide the best measures to employ in order for the delivery system to function as it was intended, working around the inevitability of settling. In general, this is a question of whether to try to keep the suspensoid dispersed as long as possible, or to allow it to settle, but control the structure the particles assume once they settle.

Formation of a cake (sediment)

The dilemma for dealing with suspensions then can become the 'redispersability' of the sedimented particles. Once settled on the bottom of a container, particles threaten to crystallize, creating a dense cake or aggregate (the 'compact' settling) that can be extremely difficult to redisperse. Some of the choices described above pertain to early stages in the sedimentation process and involve manipulation of sedimentation velocity (v). Though it may seem counterintuitive, it actually may be advantageous either to increase or decrease sedimentation velocity, depending on the ultimate system design. If suspension particles are more dense than the suspension medium, they are destined to settle into a structured crystalline cake. What parameters influencing crystal growth come into play once a suspension has settled? Two include temperature fluctuations and Ostwald ripening.

Recall in Chapter 3 it was said that all materials are soluble to some extent in a given solvent. A suspension's behavior can be viewed as a dispersion of a solid in a saturated solution. Temperature fluctuations then can affect this nominal 'solubility.' The outcome is dependent on the heat of solution, ΔH_{soln}. When the insoluble particles settle to the bottom of the container, forming a dense cake, crystal bridges between particles can develop. Crystallization starts with one particle, then bridges to others. Using this 'saturated solution' model, the effect of temperature on crystal growth is illustrated with the van't Hoff equation:

$$\ln\frac{S_2}{S_1} = \frac{\Delta H_{soln}}{R}\left[\frac{(T_2 - T_1)}{(T_1 T_2)}\right]$$

where

S_1 = solubility (i.e., $g \cdot mL^{-1}$) at temperature T_1
S_2 = solubility at temperature T_2
ΔH_{soln} = heat of solution ($cal \cdot mol^{-1}$)
$R = 1.99 \; cal \cdot mol^{-1}$
T = temperature (K).

When rearranged to focus on solubility, the form is:

$$S_2 = S_1 e^{\left(\frac{\Delta H_{soln}}{R} \left[\frac{(T_2 - T_1)}{(T_1 T_2)} \right] \right)}$$

When ΔH_{soln} is positive, which is true when $S_2 > S_1$, the 'solubility' increases with increasing temperature. Adding heat to the system, moving from T_1 to T_2, increases solubility, from S_1 to S_2. When ΔH_{soln} is negative, which is true when $S_1 < S_2$, solubility decreases with increasing temperature, so adding heat to the system will decrease solubility. What does this mean? First, that solubility is a function of the heat of solution, so temperature can positively or negatively influence the degree of solubility viewed here in a thermodynamic way. Second, that variation in temperature causes transient increases and decreases in 'solubility'. By changing S, especially with several fluctuations, more opportunities arise for particles to sediment, and once it begins, simply returning to an initial temperature does not guarantee reversal of crystallization. Temperature fluctuations can initiate and accelerate crystal growth within the sediment.

Key Point

> Two important components regarding suspension caking include temperature fluctuations and crystal growth via Ostwald ripening.

Ostwald ripening is a process by which particles that do arise, such as those from temperature fluctuations, tend to become larger and tend to deposit on progressively larger particles at the expense of smaller particles. This process of creating larger particles is thermodynamically favored over retention of small particles because small crystals have a larger surface area-to-volume ratio than do large crystals. Ostwald ripening is described by the Kelvin equation (also called the Ostwald–Freundlich equation):

$$RT \ln \left[\frac{P}{P_0} \right] = \left[\frac{2\gamma v}{r} \right]$$

where

P = vapor pressure over a curved surface
P_0 = vapor pressure over a flat surface
γ = interfacial free energy
v = molar volume
r = radius
$R = 8.314 \times 10^7$ erg/mol K
$T = 298$ (K).

The Kelvin equation pertains to boundaries between two phases, relating surface tension of a boundary with its curvature. It tells us that vapor pressure over a curved surface is greater than over a less curved surface. Smaller spheres have increased curvature, and so increased vapor pressure (escaping tendency). How does this relate to the dispersed phase particles? Stated in another way, small particles have better 'solubility' than large particles. So, small particles disappear and larger particles grow at the expense of the small particles. This is not a 'thermal' process – it cannot be avoided even under conditions of constant temperature. The result pertinent to suspensions is that this process leads to caking. Caking is dense packing of particles through formation of rigid structure.

So, to summarize, considering both the van't Hoff and Kelvin equations, it can be gathered that a major obstacle to maintaining usefulness of suspensions is the reinforcement, or amplification, of the strength of interparticulate cohesion, especially at distances in the range of closer PE minima (i.e., intermolecular interactions). These, in turn can be temperature-fluctuation dependent.

Conceding the inevitable: Management versus avoidance

As mentioned previously, when settling occurs, the dosage form is not necessarily ruined if the conditions under which the particles settle are controlled. What can be done to ensure the settled suspensoid (particles) can be reconstituted with reasonable effort? First, it must be conceded that 'interactions' among components of complex pharmaceutical suspensions are predestined. However, there are choices of how to exert some control over sedimentation, depending on what is most suitable for the particular delivery system. The two potential courses of action include: 1) attempting to avoid suspensoid interactions or 2) trying to manage the interactions. Ultimately, the goal of either path is to keep the suspension delivery system usable. Avoidance has the aim of precluding, or at least delaying, suspensoid interactions. Management has the aim of optimizing the way in which the suspensoid settles. First, two terms must be defined. Flocculation is the creation of floccules. Floccules are flakes, or loose, irregularly shaped particles. When they settle they do not compact well. Deflocculation, then, is the antithesis: the intentional creation of a coagulated system. Though deflocculation may sound counterproductive, there are some situations when it is the better alternative. Variations of either extreme are also commonly employed.

Flocculation and deflocculation

Creation of a flocculated system is the approach to precluding or delaying interactions among the components of a suspension and can involve use of a structured vehicles to slow sedimentation rate (velocity). Deflocculation is intentional coagulation of the system and also can employ structured vehicles.

I. Flocculation

Flocculation is a method of prohibiting settled particles from creating a structured crystalline cake so that they exist as loose aggregates. Flocculation is achieved by creating charge and/or stearic irregularities on the surfaces of suspension particles (causing them to act as 'flakes' or 'fluff'), while retaining some repulsive energy between particles. The goal is to force irregular packing of the particles when they settle, with large interparticulate distances, allowing weak attractive interactions among the particles. The attractive interactions are weak enough to allow for physical redispersion to be possible. Flocculation can be used to resist the compression, induced by gravity, borne by suspended particles. Intentionally causing flocculation of a suspension is one method by which resuspendability can be ensured.

Recall from Chapter 6 the PE of interaction in dispersions, $V_T = V_A + V_R + V_S$, where V_T = total interaction energy, V_A = van der Waals attractive energy, V_R = electrostatic repulsion via the electrical double layer, and V_S = steric and solvent repulsion. Also recall that repulsive forces are shorter-range than are attractive forces (Figure 7.4), which creates two PE minima that are energetically favorable separation distances for particles to occupy. The discussion in Chapter 6 was in regard to colloidal dispersions, but the concepts are also applicable to suspensions.

The outer PE minimum (approximately 1000–2000 Å apart) is where successful flocculation holds loosely aggregated particles and the inner PE minimum is where coagulation is likely to occur. If particles are held at the 'flocculation'

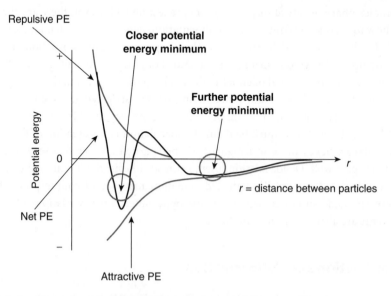

Figure 7.4 Two potential energy (PE) minima where particles may reside

Particles with a separation distance at the outer energy minimum have the smallest PE of the two minima, and so are more easily redispersed than those that are separated by the distance denoted by the closer PE minimum.

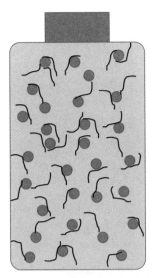

Figure 7.5 Flocculated suspension with or without a suspending agent

Sedimentation is minimized; accomplished using electrolytes (to decrease zeta potential) or addition of polymers, illustrated here by extensions from the particles (steric hindrance, etc.) or surfactants. *(Not drawn to scale.)*

minimum, it can be seen by comparing the PEs, redispersion of the suspensoid is less energetically demanding and more likely to be feasible than for particles that have moved to the coagulation energy well. So, when it is decided a suspension should be stabilized by flocculation, the goal is to direct the particles to the outer PE well where they will hopefully remain. Figure 7.5 illustrates the concept of a flocculated suspension.

The potential drawback of flocculated suspensions is their rapid rate of separation (rising or falling), leaving a distinct boundary between the sediment and the dispersion medium. This can appear unsightly, but the most significant detractor may be the necessity to use the dispersion quickly after agitation or risk inaccuracies in measurement of dispersed system. Three potential outcomes of flocculate volume that can result from flocculation include volumes that are less than, equal to or greater than the original dispersion volume, as represented in Figure 7.6.

How is flocculation achieved? Flocculation is the creation of large interparticulate distances, so that only weak net attractive interactions (molecular interactions) among dispersed phase particles are allowed. Those interactions that are allowed to occur should be easily broken when the delivery system is agitated. There are three general methods by which flocculation is accomplished: electrolyte addition, use of polymers and use of surfactants.

Flocculation by electrolyte addition

Just as can occur with colloidal dispersions, addition of electrolytes (counterions to charged surface) to suspensions can decrease the repulsion between like surface

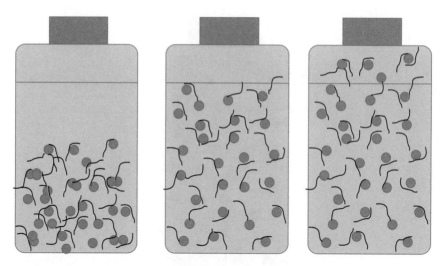

Figure 7.6 Three potential outcomes of flocculation

The flocculate volume can be less than, equal to, or greater than the original dispersion volume. The clear supernatant (left) or excess volume (right) are acceptable from a performance standpoint, but can be considered unsightly. To create a more elegant suspension, the center suspension illustrates an ideal product.

charges. Depending on the surface charge on the particle surface either cationic or anionic electrolytes are employed. Since the Debye length $(1/K)$ is compromised by the square of the counterion valence, polyvalent counterions are the most effective electrolyte flocculating agents. Cationic flocculating agents (for negatively charged surfaces) are (preferably) polyvalent cations, such as Al^{3+} from the addition of aluminum chloride. A useful anionic flocculating agent is sodium sulfate (useful for the SO_4^{2-}).

Flocculation by polymer addition

Long chain hydrophilic colloids can be employed to physically keep suspensoid particles separated in hydrophilic dispersion media. These are typically long-chain, high molecular weight compounds with active groups spaced along their length. Part of the chain adsorbs onto the suspended particle surface, while part extends out into dispersion medium, forming loose bridges that provide controlled distances between suspensoid particles (Figure 7.7). An example of a flocculating polymer is gelatin. It should be noted that, with either electrolyte or polymer flocculation, changes in pH can reverse the advantages imparted by the flocculating agent.

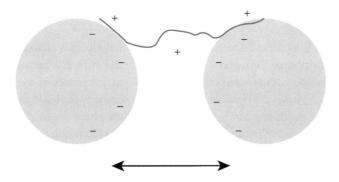

Figure 7.7 Polymer flocculation

A positively charged colloid is adsorbed onto negative suspensoid particles, and keeps them from getting any closer. In this illustration, the active groups contained in the polymer are positively charged.

Flocculation using surfactants

Surfactants (both ionic and nonionic) are sometimes useful as flocculating agents because of their ability to decrease zeta potential, facilitating the initial dispersion of the suspensoid. In addition, nonionic surfactants can act as polymer flocculating agents, especially at high concentrations.

II. Deflocculation

Deflocculated (coagulated) systems allow the dispersed phase to proceed to the outer PE minimum, while retaining their existence as separate particles. Gravity threatens to overcome the interparticulate repulsive forces, which can result in compression of the dispersed phase into a dense sediment that is difficult or impossible to redisperse. In contrast to flocculated systems, deflocculated suspensions often have no clear boundary between phases, so they can have a pleasing appearance and they typically have slow sedimentation rates. Once they do sediment though, difficulties can arise. Deflocculated systems may require a structured vehicle to keep the dispersed phase suspended. Structured vehicles (suspending agents) can be useful for both flocculated and deflocculated systems, keeping particles apart by increasing η, the viscosity of the dispersion medium, thereby decreasing the rate of suspensoid particle interactions and sedimentation velocity. However, if viscosity is too greatly increased this can actually become an impediment to easy redispersion. Carboxymethylcellulose, microcrystalline cellulose, polyvinyl pyrrolidone, bentonite, veegum, tragacanth, carbomer, and xanthan gum can act as viscosity-imparting agents.

B. Emulsions

An emulsion is a coarse dispersion of (usually) liquid globules (100–50 000 nm in diameter) distributed throughout a liquid vehicle in which it is immiscible. More complex emulsions, composed of more than two major phases, and emulsions of other types of phases are possible. Though more complex, the basic principles still apply. Simple emulsions can be thought of as 'three-phase systems,' a two-phase system plus an emulsifying agent (surfactant). The most common emulsion delivery systems are liquids and the two major phases are both liquids. As for all disperse systems, these two phases are the internal (discontinuous) phase and the external (continuous) phase. Without the surfactant (emulsifying agent), both phases would simply separate, as occurs if oil and water are mixed, with the less dense liquid rising to the top. Separation occurs because the interfacial tension of each liquid is too great to allow the liquids to mix. The emulsifier keeps the liquids from separating by decreasing interfacial tension between the two major phases. Recall many surfactants are amphiphiles and so possess solubility in both phases of an emulsion. Liquid emulsions may be either 'oil-in-water' (O/W) or 'water-in-oil (W/O).' These are dispersions of oil in an aqueous continuous phase or dispersions of water in an oily continuous phase, respectively (Figure 7.8). If the emulsifying agent acts correctly, the result is a dispersion of one liquid in the other.

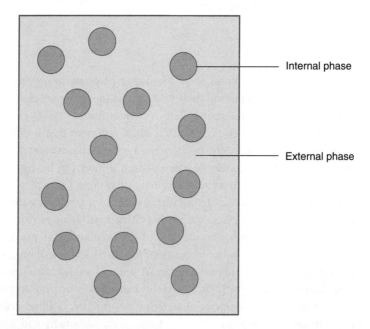

Figure 7.8 Representation of an emulsion

Depending on the emulsion type, the internal (discontinuous) and external (continuous) phases can be either aqueous or oily, but not similar to each other.

If the droplets (in Figure 7.8) are oil-based, the continuous phase is aqueous and the emulsion is called an O/W emulsion. If the droplets are aqueous, a W/O emulsion exists.

Key Point

An emulsion takes on the physical characteristics of its external or continuous phase.

Key Point

An emulsion requires an emulsifying agent and work input in order to be created.

The first general rule for emulsions is that the emulsion takes on the characteristics of the external (continuous) phase, i.e., the emulsion will feel, smell, taste, and appear to be whichever phase is external. The second rule is that, without the emulsifying agent and some work input, the thermodynamics of a two-phase system favor coalescence of each liquid separately. That is, the lowest PE possible for the system as a whole would be for the liquids to be separate, with the lowest possible interfacial tensions. Even if work (agitation or stirring) is applied, there is nothing to keep the dissimilar constituents dispersed in one another in the absence of a surfactant (Figure 7.9). After agitation, though dispersed, the liquids are at high PEs and will move to lower PE states (separation) if not hindered. Thus, as with most disperse systems, emulsions are naturally thermodynamically unstable because the dispersed liquid is held at an intermediate potential energy, but this is not as low PE as complete separation.

Even with energy input (shear), the system illustrated in Figure 7.9 will return to its original state once the shear is removed. If a surfactant is added, the interfacial tension between the two disparate liquids is decreased. The liquids can then reach a reasonably stable state, as an emulsion. In this case, the phase that coalesces fastest will tend to be the external phase. In addition to its overt interfacial actions, a surfactant plays a major role with regard to which phase is favored for more rapid coalescence, and so can dictate which phase is the external phase of an emulsion. How fast will a phase coalesce? The coalescence speed – or rate – of a liquid 'x' is represented by the equation below. In general, the rate a liquid will coalesce is proportional to its relative concentration and innate PE barriers that are characteristic of the specific liquid, and is inversely proportional to temperature:

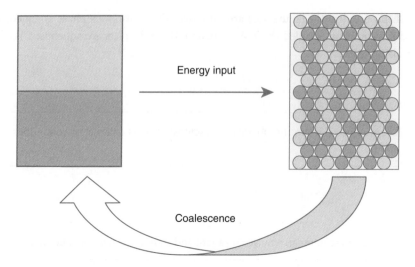

Figure 7.9 Energy input temporarily mixes two immiscible liquids

The system as displayed on the left has overall lower potential energy (PE) than in the mixed state (right). Energy input, such as stirring or other form of agitation will temporarily cause mixing of immiscible liquids. When mixed, the liquids gain PE. When energy input is discontinued, the two liquids will separate and revert to their initial conditions, as separate liquids, at lower PE. In other words, if work in the form of agitation or stirring is applied, two immiscible liquids (left) will temporarily mix (right) but the mixture is thermodynamically unstable. To regain stability, the less dense liquid (usually an oil) will return to its normal orientation above the more dense liquid (usually aqueous), and return to its original state (left).

$$\text{Rate}_x = C_x e^{\frac{-W_x}{RT}}$$

where

Rate_x = rate of droplet coalescence
C_x = collision frequency factor for droplets
W_x = energy barrier to droplet coalescence

Key Point

The phase that coalesces the fastest will tend to be the external phase of an emulsion.

A qualitative inspection of the equation reveals that, the greater the number of collisions (C_x), the more likely the liquid is to coalesce. Energy barriers to coalescence include parameters such as droplet viscosity, surface tension, electrostatic repulsion between particles and effects of shear created by agitation of the system. The greater the barrier(s) hindering collisions (W_x), the more C_x is opposed. Barriers to collision include viscosity of the other liquid, electrical repulsion between droplets, any hydration layer that must be overcome for coalescence to occur and the fraction of the interface covered by the emulsifying agent. Thus, the coalescence rates of the two phases work in opposite directions: one toward coalescing the aqueous phase and one toward coalescing the oily phase.

The 'barriers' to coalescence have been discussed to some degree above, in the previous section and previous chapters, with regard to their actions that oppose coalescence. If a viscosity-increasing agent is added to either phase, it will slow the mobility of that phase and promote slower coalescence of that phase, and so the tendency will be for the more viscous phase to become the internal phase. If a phase is protected by a hydration sheath, the protection must be ruptured before coalescence can occur, which slows coalescence. Electrical repulsion between individual droplets has been discussed with regard to colloidal dispersions and suspensions, but it also applies to emulsions.

The coalescence barrier not yet discussed is that of the emulsifying agent. The larger the fraction of the interface covered by the emulsifying agent, the more tightly packed around the interface are the molecules of the emulsifying agent, and the greater the barrier to coalescence of the coated phase. Therefore, resolution of the two rates can depend solely on the relative solubility of an emulsifying agent in each phase. Bancroft's rule states that the phase in which the emulsifying agent is more soluble tends to become the external phase of that emulsion.

Key Point

Bancroft's rule states that the phase in which an emulsifying agent is more soluble tends to become the external (continuous) phase of the resulting emulsion.

Figures 7.10 and 7.11 illustrate the effects described by Bancroft's rule, using an amphiphile as an emulsifying agent. Solubility of an emulsifying agent can also result in changes in the physical proximity particles can assume, depending on the nature of the emulsifier. Altering the composition – or balance – of an amphiphile can impart important differences in resulting emulsions. Amphiphiles, therefore, can be assigned a hydrophilic lipophilic balance (HLB) number. The larger the assigned HLB, the more hydrophilic in nature is the amphiphile (see Chapter 5).

Figure 7.10 is an illustration of a hypothetical amphiphile. This amphiphile can be synthesized such that its composition favors solubility in either oil or water, as desired. An amphiphile that is predominantly lipophilic is illustrated in Figure 7.11. Possessing a lipophilic-predominant composition, it is more soluble in lipid than water, and this characteristic influences which phase will be the external phase (oil), and so the type of emulsion formed.

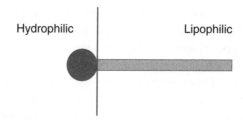

Figure 7.10 Amphiphile emulsifying agent and two phases

This amphiphile is drawn to indicate it has better solubility in oil than water (by representing a larger portion of the molecule labeled 'lipophilic').

A.

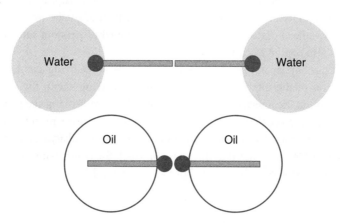

B.

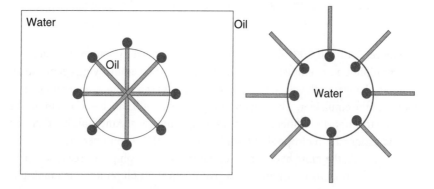

Figure 7.11 Emulsifying agent solubility (monomolecular film formation)

In (A), the amphiphile has greater solubility in oil than water. This would provide a tendency for water-in-oil emulsions to form (above) as the 'particles' of oil (lower) are able to approach each other more closely than those of water (above), increasing the likelihood oil will be the external phase. The potential dispersed phase molecules can be visualized (B).

Potential problems encountered with emulsions include creaming, sedimentation, aggregation, and coalescence, and all reflect the basic thermodynamic instability inherent with emulsions. Creaming is the upward movement of dispersed droplets relative to the continuous phase, whereas sedimentation is the downward movement of dispersed droplets. Aggregation (flocculation) occurs when dispersed droplets come together but do not fuse. This is the same action described previously for suspensions as a means of adding control over the suspensions. Whether an emulsion tends toward creaming or sedimentation depends on the nature of the emulsion (O/W or W/O). Coalescence (also called cracking) is complete fusion of the droplets. Creaming and sedimentation of emulsions, like sedimentation of suspensions, is inevitable (and analogous to sedimentation of suspensions). The destabilized droplets follow behavior described by Stokes' law. Creaming, sedimentation, aggregation, and coalescence are undesirable but often reversible. However, as with all disperse systems, degradation can be permanent. Physical pharmacy issues regarding emulsions originate from intermolecular interactions and follow parameters defined in previous discussion.

Stokes' law applies to emulsions as well as suspensions and many of the problems occurring with emulsions can be improved utilizing the same types of approaches used with other disperse systems. (Keep in mind, since emulsions may cream or sediment, the sign of velocity, v, in Stokes' law indicates direction of movement and can be negative or positive.) The smaller the dispersed phase droplets, the slower creaming or sedimentation (velocity, rising or falling) will occur. Consider manipulations of emulsion systems that might be anticipated through Stokes' law. Adding viscosity-inducing agents to the continuous phase increases η of the continuous phase, after the emulsion is formed, can slow movement of the dispersed phase (either up or down), and so can be helpful in some situations. Perhaps the density difference between the phases ($\rho_{\text{dispersed phase}} - \rho_{\text{dispersion medium}}$) can be reduced. The emulsified droplet size, r, can sometimes be varied (e.g., microemulsions).

Three types of emulsifying agents

The type of emulsifying agent employed can also affect the stability of an emulsion. There are three types of emulsifying agents: monomolecular film formers, multimolecular film formers, and solid particle films. Emulsifiers act either by lowering interfacial tension or by forming a protective barrier that physically resists coalescence. Each will be briefly discussed.

I. Monomolecular film formers

Monomolecular film formers (as depicted in Figures 7.11 and 7.12) are the most common emulsifying agents, are very versatile, and are surfactants (they locate at

A. **Anionic**

Sodium dodecyl sulfate

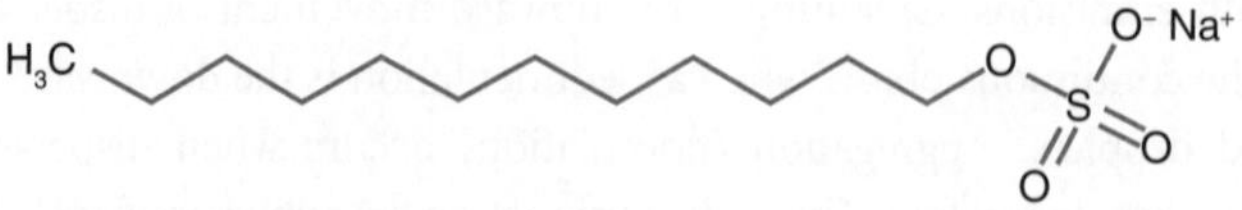

Sodium dioctylsulfosuccinate

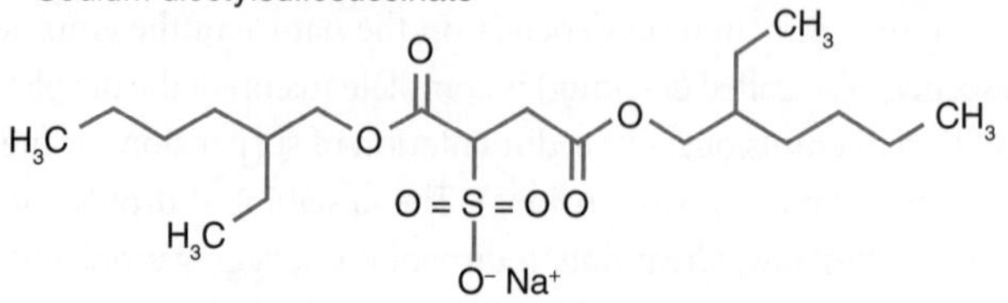

B. **Cationic**

Cetrimide

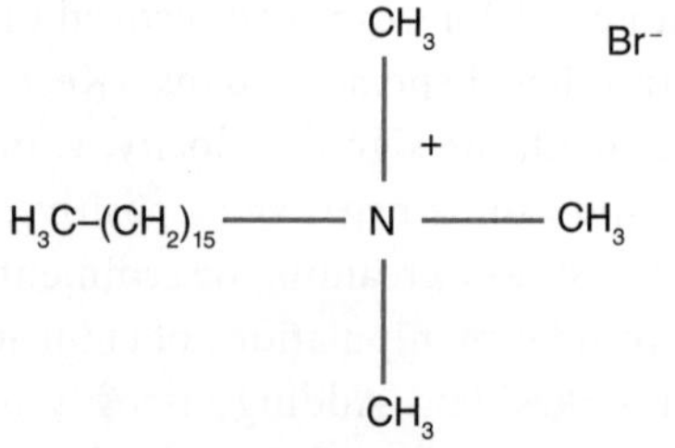

cetrimide
(cetrimonium bromide)
$C_{19}H_{42}NBr$

Cetylpyridinium chloride

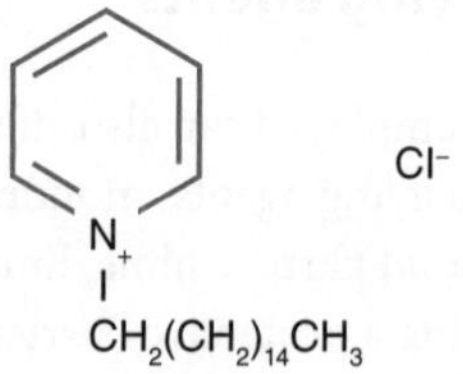

C. **Nonionic**

Glyceryl monostearate

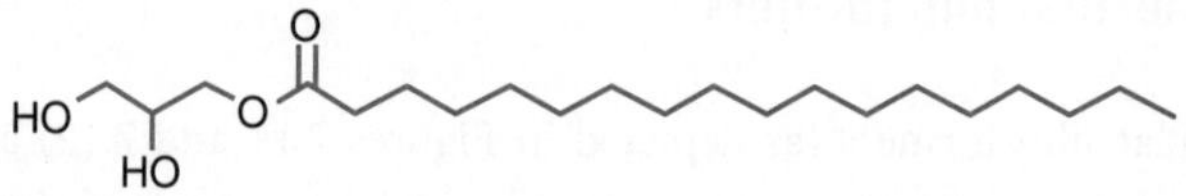

Polyoxyethylene sorbitan monostearate (Tween 60)

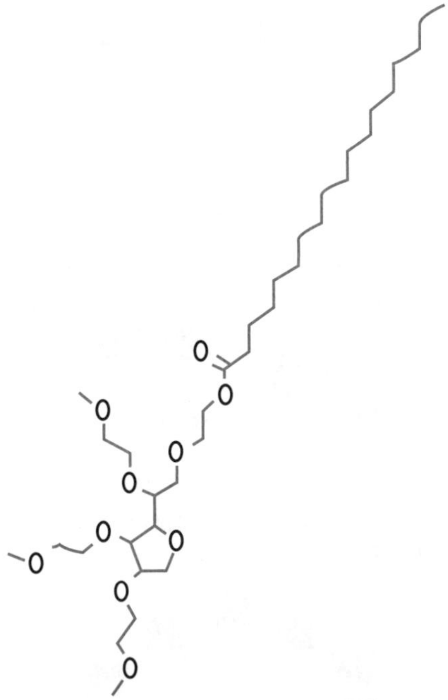

Figure 7.12 The three types of film-forming emulsifying agents

In this figure, an oil-in-water emulsion is used to consider how each of the three film-forming emulsifying agents act at the oil droplet–water dispersion medium interface. Each of the types of monomolecular film-forming emulsifiers is illustrated, with two examples of each. Cationic agents impart a positive charge to the dispersed droplet surface, while anionic agents impart negative charges. These charges add to the protection of the dispersed droplets. Nonionic agents do not impart additional charge to the dispersed droplets, but still offer physical protection.

an interface because of their amphiphilic character). They form single layers (monomolecular layers) around the dispersed phase particles and this single layer resists coalescence. Monomolecular film forming emulsifiers are used to lower interfacial tension (decrease coalescence barriers, 'W') and may be ionized on the hydrophilic portion of the agent. Ionization of an emulsifying agent can add stability to the emulsion by adding charge repulsion. Monomolecular film forming emulsifiers then can be anionic, cationic, zwitterioinic, or nonionic types. The preceding illustrations of amphiphilic molecules are part of this category of emulsifying agents. Examples of anionic, cationic, and nonionic surfactants are shown in Figure 7.12.

II. Multimolecular film formers

Multimolecular film formers (Figure 7.13) usually are hydrophilic colloids used to coat the internal phase (several layers thick) – which is more commonly the oily

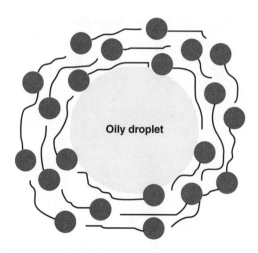

Figure 7.13   A multimolecular film forming emulsifying agent

Hydrophilic colloids can be utilized to coat the internal phases of oil-in-water emulsions, forming a physical, not interfacial, barrier to coalescence.

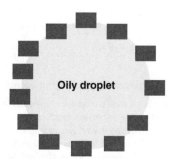

Figure 7.14   A solid particle film emulsifying agent

Solid particles can be used to create a film around the internal phases of emulsions, forming a physical barrier to coalescence.

phase. This physically imparts resistance to coalescence due to the thick, sometimes charged, layer surrounding each oily droplet, providing stability to these types of emulsions. A second action these agents possess is the ability to swell, increasing dispersion medium viscosity, further preventing dispersed phase droplets from coalescing. Note multimolecular film formers do not usually appreciably lower interfacial tension, but rather make a physical barrier to coalescence. Examples of multimolecular film forming emulsifying agents include acacia, tragacanth, gelatin, methylcellulose, and polyethylene glycols.

III. Solid particle films

Solid particle films (Figure 7.13), like multimolecular film formers, are also simply physical barriers to coalescence, and so do not act via interfacial tension. They must have some degree of both lipid and aqueous solubility in order to remain at the interface. This type of emulsifying agent employs adsorption of finely divided solid particles to the surfaces of the internal phase of emulsions, creating particulate films. The particles must be small, relative to the dispersed droplet size – meaning, usually colloidal in size – but this appears to be the major defining parameter of this class of emulsifying agents as it is possible any solid could be a candidate. The particles have areas of high and low PE, and so can be wetted by both polar and nonpolar phases. Importantly, they can be collected by droplets of the dispersed phase. Either O/W or W/O emulsions can be created with the same agents. In addition, most solid particle emulsifying agents also swell in the dispersion medium, increasing its viscosity – decreasing collision frequency of dispersed droplets. Examples of solid particle film emulsifying agents include bentonite, veegum, and aluminum hydroxide.

Summary

Like fine dispersions, the rules that apply to coarse dispersions are largely based on particle–particle attraction, repulsion, and movement. Dispersions, in general, are often relatively unstable – some more than others. The instability is due to overall thermodynamic drive toward conditions of lowest PE. When we utilize disperse systems, we often must proactively include in the system mechanisms that will inhibit or slow progress from higher PE to lower. Failure to do so often results in such stable, but useless situations, where enormous amounts of energy – or work – would be required to re-establish a usable drug delivery system. Prevention is usually the track taken, via methods aimed at inhibiting excessive interparticulate interactions. Planning ahead, by creating artificial PE 'holding points' is another approach.

Coarse dispersions include suspensions and emulsions, which generally have larger dispersed phase particles or droplets than do colloids. Suspensions (for this text) are systems in which solid particles are dispersed in a liquid. In contrast, the most common emulsions encountered in drug delivery systems are liquid droplets dispersed in a liquid. For all coarse dispersions, the dispersed phase does not naturally disperse, and especially, it does not remain dispersed in its dispersion medium. These systems ultimately will resist these conditions. But these often are the conditions under which our dosage form is useful. Therefore, methods must be utilized that either prevent coarse dispersions from aggregating and coagulating – conditions most energetically favorable – or allow partial movement to aggregation and coagulation with a 'stop point' near the lowest PE well that will allow us to recreate the dispersion when we want to use it, without employing an inordinate effort. To avoid aggregation, we can affect the viscosity, pH, electrolyte concentration, temperature, and particle size of both the dispersed phase and dispersion medium. To prepare a coarse dispersion so that we can later redisperse it, we can create predetermined conditions of pH or add components that resist tight packing of the aggregate.

Coarse dispersions are useful for approximating the actions of solutions when the dispersed particles are not soluble in the dispersion media. Advantage can be taken of the internal phase of coarse dispersions by placing otherwise insoluble or unpalatable components of the dosage form within the dispersed phase – and away from the dispersion medium. Coarse dispersions, however, are prone to destabilizing conditions, and so elements, such as dispersion media ionic strength, pH, temperature and temperature fluctuations, among other parameters, must be carefully controlled.

Self-assessment questions

1. What is a coarse dispersion?

2. What are suspensions and how do they differ from other liquid drug delivery systems?

3. What are emulsions and how do they differ from other liquid drug delivery systems?

4. What is the approximate size of suspension and emulsion dispersed phase particles, and how does this differ from particle sizes of other liquid delivery systems?

5. Why is sedimentation of a suspension so undesirable?

6. What is flocculation? How are floccules created?

7. Using Stokes' law, what can we alter that can help or harm coarse dispersions by separation and coagulation?

8. Why do we want particles and droplets of coarse dispersions to reside at distances of the outer PE minima?

9. What is Bancroft's rule?

10. What are the three classes of emulsifying agents?

Answers to self-assessment questions

Chapter 1

Q1. Intermolecular interactions, mainly those of attraction, cause molecules to act with more restriction when they are in proximity to each other. This is the case with condensed phases, such as liquids. The attraction among molecules is much greater in liquids than in gasses, resulting in great differences in measureable criteria, such as vapor pressure. Adhesive and cohesive forces cause this.

Q2. Forces of attraction between the two different molecules should be greater than between similar molecules.

Q3. From intramolecular interactions.

Q4. Dipole–induced dipole interactions.

Q5. The three main intermolecular interactions that pertain to pure liquids include dipole–dipole, dipole–induced dipole and induced dipole–induced dipole interactions.

Q6. Attractive forces are van der Waals forces. Repulsive forces are electrostatic forces.

Q7. Adhesive forces are forces of attraction between dissimilar substances. Cohesive forces are forces of attraction between similar substances.

Q8. Polarity is the tendency of a molecule to form dipoles. Polarizability is the ease with which dipole moments can be created, or induced, in a molecule. If two liquids with similar polarity or polarizability, α, are combined, the closer the polarizabilities of the two are, the better they will tend to mix. Polarizability is a measurable quantity, and so thoughtful use of this quantity can assist with creating stable drug delivery systems.

Q9. Dipole–dipole, dipole–induced dipole, induced dipole–induced dipole, ion–dipole and ion–induced dipole. The larger the dipole moment, μ, the greater the attractive force among molecules of a pure liquid. When considering adding one liquid to another, matching liquid dipole moments will tend to provide miscible combinations.

Q10. Energy is required to separate molecules. The highest energy requirement occurs when a system (a mixture of substances) is at a potential energy (PE) minimum, meaning it is very stable. If there arises the need to separate components of the system, it can be very difficult to overcome the large PE.

Chapter 2

Q1. A material capable of dissolving another, forming a solution.

Q2. Water is considered a polar solvent, acetone a semipolar solvent and olive oil a nonpolar solvent. Water would be the best of the three.

Q3. Again, water would be expected to be the better solvent, this time because of its relatively higher dielectric constant.

Q4. Polar solvents utilize strong dipoles and hydrogen bonding. They work mostly through dipole–dipole and dipole–induced dipole interactions, mixing with other polar molecules, including those with –OH groups.

Semipolar solvents also utilize strong dipoles, but lack hydrogen bonding. They work through dipole–dipole and dipole–induced dipole interactions, mixing with polar and other semipolar molecules, including those with lower dielectric constants.

Nonpolar solvents have little or no dipole. They work through induced dipole–induced dipole interactions, mixing with other nonpolar substances, such as oils and fats.

Q5. The dielectric constant is the ratio of the capacitance of a material compared to the capacitance of a reference, usually air, and is used to measure how much electrostatic energy the substance can store.

Q6. Matching materials with similar dielectric constants enhances the likelihood they will mix.

Q7. Yes, because the relatively high dielectric constant of glycerin compared to calcium sulfate allows glycerin to pull the ionic bonds of calcium sulfate apart. The true solubility (at 15°C) is 5.2 g calcium sulfate/100 g glycerin.

Q8. $0.10(\varepsilon_{glycerin}) + 0.90(\varepsilon_{water}) = 0.10(47.0 \text{ F/m}) + 0.90(80.4 \text{ F/m}) = 4.7 + 72.4 = 77.1 \text{ F/m}.$

Q9. To dissolve – or make solutions with – various substances needed for drug delivery systems, when those substances cannot be given to patients in their natural state.

Q10. Polar. Nonpolar solvents are those with dielectric constants (and so will dissolve substance with dielectric constants) of 1–20. Semipolar solvents are best for dielectric constants of 20–50, and polar solvents for dielectric constants above 50. With an estimated dielectric constant of 77.1, the mixture would be a polar solvent, best used for polar solutes.

Chapter 3

Q1. A solution is a combination of at least two materials that are dissolved, meaning the solute is dispersed on a molecular level in the solvent.

Q2. Solubility is the final quantity of solute that will dissolve in a solvent. Dissolution is the action that occurs up to the endpoint of solubility.

Q3. By choosing a solvent best suited to the characteristics of the solute, such as polar with polar, or nonpolar with nonpolar. Also, increasing solute surface area (by decreasing particle size), altering the temperature (perhaps increasing or decreasing), and perhaps changing the pH of the solvent to increase the ionization of the solute.

Q4. Seen through the Noyes–Whitney equation, possibly helpful would be increased diffusion through increased stirring and making the particle size smaller.

Q5. Disintegration, deaggregation, and dissolution.

Q6. Wetting, immersion, and diffusion.

Q7. $0°$.

Q8. An agent that reduces surface or interfacial tension, allowing particle wetting and possibly mixing.

Q9. A mathematical model that relates solute concentration gradient and diffusion layer surrounding a solute particle to dissolution rate.

Q10. In order for wetting to occur, the work of adhesion must exceed the work of cohesion (adhesion must exceed cohesion).

Chapter 4

Q1. Colligative means it has to do with the number of particles rather than the nature of the particles. A colligative property is one that is affected by the number of particles in solution, not what the particles actually are.

Q2. Vapor pressure, boiling point, freezing point, and osmotic pressure of the solvent. The four standard equations commonly used are:

Vapor pressure lowering $\Delta P = X_2 P_1$
Boiling point elevation $\Delta T_b = K_b m$
Freezing point depression $\Delta T_f = K_f m$
Osmotic pressure (elevation) $\Pi = RTm$.

Q3. Because these correction values help account for incorrectly assuming complete solute dissociation where ionization occurs.

Q4. Colligative properties help us quantify changes in tonicity of solutions. Many tissues of the body have small ability to withstand tonicity outside of certain tolerances without being damaged. Therefore, by observing colligative properties we can prepare isotonic solutions.

Q5. Exerting the same pressure as another substance. In the case of solutions, exerting the same osmotic pressure against membranes as physiological solutions.

Q6. It is diffusion, and lack of it, through a membrane that causes tonicity. Some solvents and solutes diffuse through a given membrane, while others cannot. This disparity causes membrane tone – or tonicity.

Q7. The individual membrane that is affected dictates the tonicity we wish to achieve. This is relatively standard for biological systems. What we are controlling is the number of particles allowed in our solutions. Molality provides us with the number of particles. Diffusion is also a part of tonicity. The Morse equation, Fick's law, and the Stokes–Einstein equation relate diffusion to surface area and thickness of the membrane, and solute concentration gradient. These, in turn, are related to particle size, solution viscosity, and temperature of the solution.

Q8. Sodium chloride is a ubiquitous salt in biology and plays a large role in natural tonicity, along with many other biological salts, proteins, and glycoproteins. Sodium chloride is so central that it is logical to use this common substance as a reference for tonicity calculations.

Q9. To make isotonic only with sodium chloride: (500 mL) × (0.90 g/100 mL) = 4.50 g NaCl

  a. 1% sodium salicylate = (1g/100 mL) × (500 mL) = 5.00 g sodium salicylate

  b. Sodium chloride equivalent of 5.00 g sodium salicylate: (5.00 g) × (0.36) = 1.80 g NaCl represented by sodium salicylate.

  c. Amount of NaCl still required: (4.50 g) – (1.80 g) = 2.70 g NaCl

Q10.

  a. g of drug in solution: (3 g/100 mL) × 15 mL = 0.45 g

  b. V value of ephedrine hydrochloride = 10.0 mL water needed to make 1 g ephedrine hydrochloride isotonic.

    Or, $V = w \times E \times 111.1$: $V =$ (0.45 g $CaCl_2$)(0.10g NaCl/1 g ephedrine hydrochloride)(111.1 mL isotonic solution/1 g NaCl) = 4.99 mL water is made isotonic with ephedrine hydrochloride.

  c. Preparation is 0.45 g ephedrine hydrochloride + (15 – 4.99 = 10.01 mL water) + (10.0 mL × 0.9 g/100 mL = 0.09 g NaCl).

Chapter 5

Q1. Typically, a surface is a boundary between a substance and air.

Q2. Differing subtly from the definition of a surface, an interface is the boundary between two substances.

Q3. Surface tension is the inward pull, into the bulk, away from air. Interfacial tension is the resulting pull into each substance's own bulk, modified by the pull into each other's bulk.

Q4. To improve wetting of solids, and thus dissolution; also, to decrease the pull into respective bulk by two disparate substances, enhancing their likelihood of mixing, even if dissimilar, to some degree.

Q5. HLB is the hydrophilic lipophilic balance number, which is an arbitrary number used to designate relative water solubility of a substance. Lower HLB numbers indicate poor water solubility, whereas higher numbers indicate better water solubility. The HLB is useful for estimating which potential dispersion media and surfactants to use in a drug delivery system, either to facilitate solid dissolution or enhance dispersions of suspensions and emulsions.

Q6. The drive to reduce the system's free energy results in a configuration that will have the minimum surface area. A sphere is the geometrical shape with minimum surface area per a given volume. A smaller surface area provides smaller interfacial energy.

Q7. Surface tension derives from the cohesive interactions of molecules in a phase. Water is polar, and the intermolecular interactions between polar molecules are stronger than the interactions between nonpolar molecules (i.e., oils).

Q8. When two condensed phases are in contact, there is more of an interaction 'across' the interface than that which exists between a condensed phase and a gas.

Q9. Surfactant molecules are amphiphilic, meaning they contain both hydrophilic and hydrophobic regions. Therefore, amphiphiles tend to locate in a way to minimize free energy of the system.

Q10. The resulting HLB is 7, which falls in the 'wetting agent' category.

Chapter 6

Q1. A system composed of heterogeneous substances, which, though one is dispersed in the other, are not solute and solvent. No dissolution is involved.

Q2. Colloids are not solutions but are fine dispersions – most often in drug delivery systems a solid dispersed in a liquid. The solid particles are smaller than those of coarse dispersions but larger than those of solutions.

Q3. Colloids contain dispersed particles 1.0–1000 nm in diameter, whereas solutes in solutions are less than 1 nm in diameter, and dispersed particles or droplets of coarse dispersions range from 100 to 50 000 nm in diameter.

Q4. They are not solutions and so are innately unstable. However, unlike coarse dispersions, colloids typically do not spontaneously separate.

Q5. Lyophobic, lyophilic, and association colloids.

Q6. This will increase N_A, and so decrease the size of the diffuse double layer (DDL, the Debye length).

Q7. Polyvalent counterions will have a much more significant effect on the thickness of the DDL than monovalent ions. Since the DDL size is related to z^2 in the equation, not only are multiple charges a consideration (polyvalent), but the effect on the DDL is squared. Increasing valence decreases the thickness of the DDL, and therefore an increased likelihood of coagulation.

Q8. This answer is not completely straightforward. It should decrease the extent of DDL. However, electrolyte concentration usually decreases dramatically (by definition, lower ε = lower electrolyte concentration), but this also decreases the value for N_A. The net effect probably will be an increased thickness of DDL, but this situation is more complicated than it might appear, so ultimately the DDL thickness can increase or decrease.

Q9. It increases the extent of the DDL. The higher kinetic energy resulting from increased temperature may overwhelm repulsive forces between dispersed phase particles. Although T is part of the numerator of the $1/K$ equation, which initially would appear to increase the extent of the DDL stabilizing the colloid, the higher kinetic energy may overwhelm repulsive force (like an egg in a frying pan) – there is more movement around and it is harder to neutralize surface charge, which can result in coagulation. It is always possible to destroy a colloid with high enough temperatures.

Q10. Always be aware of electrolyte concentrations, and especially be aware if replacing electrolytes in the dispersion medium to those with higher valences. Also, pay attention to changes in pH as some ionization will be altered in aqueous dispersions. Last, the effects of temperature sometimes are overlooked.

Chapter 7

Q1. A (usually) liquid drug delivery system with a dispersed phase larger than colloids, and typically more unstable than colloids or solutions, so tend to settle or separate. The dispersed phase is either solid or liquid.

Q2. Coarse dispersions of solid particles in liquids.

Q3. Coarse dispersions of liquid droplet in liquids. The dispersed liquid is insoluble in the dispersion medium.

Q4. Coarse dispersion dispersed phase particles or droplets are about 100–50 000 nm in diameter, which are larger than those of solutions (<1 nm) or colloids (1–1000 nm).

Q5. Sediments begin to crystalize. As the crystals grow, the sediment becomes more stable, and so harder to redisperse. The crystal growth occurs due to temperature fluctuations and Ostwald ripening.

Q6. Flocculation is the creation of loose, irregular flakes of the dispersed phase to allow easier redispersion. Floccules are created by adding electrolytes, polymers, and/or surfactants to the system.

Q7. Dispersed particle radius and dispersion medium viscosity. Perhaps dispersion medium density, if another dispersion medium is available.

Q8. Because less kinetic energy is required to recover the drug delivery system from these minima than for minima that would allow closer contact between particles/droplets.

Q9. The phase in which the emulsifying agent is most soluble tends to become the external phase of that emulsion.

Q10. Monomolecular film-formers, multimolecular film-formers, and solid particle films.

Index